YOU ARE A BETTER
PARKINSON'S DISEASE
CAREGIVER THAN YOU THINK

What Every Caregiver Should Know

KEVIN KLOS, M.D.

Forward by J. Eric Ahlskog, PhD, MD
Mayo Clinic Parkinson's Disease Specialist

For my mom, Judy Klos, as you
heroically battle this difficult condition

CONTENTS

ACKNOWLEDGMENTS

Extensive effort and time went into the research and writing of this book. In fact, this book and the research required took me more than seven years to complete due to my busy clinical practice and research schedule. My family would ask each year, "Dad, did you publish the book yet?" I am proud to now say, "Yes, the book is published!"

I would first like to thank my incredible wife, Shannon, for her loving encouragement and support. She has kept my practice running and she has kept our household running. She is a model caregiver for our beautiful seven children. I could not have completed this project without the loving support and understanding of Shannon and our seven children. Thank you for believing in me and for your unwavering love.

I would like to thank all of the patients, care partners, and caregivers who were willing to share their stories and lessons learned. A special thanks to the caregivers willing to complete exhaustive questionnaires and participate in the advisory board conferences. You have taught me far more than I have been able to teach you and for that I am deeply appreciative. Thank you for allowing me to share your insight with others. A special thank you to Joe Williams for his content editing, constructive criticism and advise on publishing this book.

I would like to thank my dear friend and colleague, Dr. Eric Ahlskog, for not only writing the foreword to this book but for all of his advice and counsel on the content and organization of this book. I am forever grateful for the mentorship and instruction that he provided me during my Neurology residency and Fellowship at the Mayo Clinic in Rochester, Minnesota. He spent countless hours sharing his knowledge and lessons learned from his over 30 years of clinical practice with me as well as guiding me on becoming a clinical researcher in Parkinson's disease. You taught me how to provide compassionate care for our patients. I am grateful for all of the years I had the opportunity to learn from such an amazing physician.

FOREWORD

It gives me great pleasure to write the foreword for this book by my good friend and colleague, Dr. Kevin Klos. Dr. Klos did his medical training at the Mayo Clinic in Rochester Minnesota. He was a neurology resident, then a Neurology Movement Disorders Fellow in our Movement Disorders Division. During those years, he saw many people with Parkinson's disease and developed superb expertise in diagnosing and managing that condition. As the Division head at that time, I strongly encouraged him to join our staff at the Mayo Clinic, and I know he thought seriously about doing this. However, his family was a strong priority and for that reason, he moved home to Oklahoma and set up a Parkinson's disease practice there. Over the years, he has been a very busy clinician and has seen countless people with Parkinson's disease. I have long contended that expertise in managing Parkinson's disease is not found in books, but rather seeing patients firsthand in the clinic. He and I both developed our clinical skills doing exactly that.

Somewhat ironically, his beloved mother has developed Parkinson's disease, giving him an added and personal perspective. We both have had substantial empathy for our patients with Parkinson's disease but the perspective of having an affected parent provides substantial, additional insight. Dr. Klos writes this book from that perspective.

Parkinson's disease is fundamentally different from many other cerebral disorders. Conditions such as strokes, encephalitis as well as most autoimmune brain conditions typically start abruptly or over days, weeks or a few months. Parkinson's disease is a neurodegenerative disorder, which starts and evolves slowly and in fact, much more slowly than most neurodegenerative conditions. Contrast Parkinson's disease to amyotrophic lateral sclerosis (Lou Gehrig's disease), which proves fatal after several years. Parkinson's disease is in distinct contrast. Note that in the current era with the available medications, people with Parkinson's disease live out a nearly normal life span. In the county in which I live (Olmsted County, Minnesota), the Parkinson's disease longevity rates are just one year short of the actuarial predictions. Fifty years ago, people with Parkinson's disease died well before their time. Hence, we have made strides although not nearly as much progress as any of us would like.

The actual duration of Parkinson's disease (PD) is much longer than most people realize. A number of subtle often symptoms start well before the movement problems that characterize typical Parkinson's disease (i.e., tremor, slowness, gait problems, etc.). PD-related conditions that may surface years or decades before the visible movement problems of Parkinson's disease include REM sleep behavior disorder (dream enactment behavior), constipation, anxiety as well as loss of the sense of smell. There are well-documented cases of one or more of these conditions surfacing 20 years or longer before the early tremor or gait problems of Parkinson's disease.

The typical movement problems characteristic of Parkinson's disease primarily relate to degeneration of a specific region in the brain called the substantia nigra. This region connects with another area of the brain called the striatum and signals there by way of neurotransmitter release. That signaling chemical of this substantia nigra-striatum connection is dopamine. Dopamine is not a common neurotransmitter in the brain. In fact, it represents less than 1% of all the brain neurotransmitters. However, it is perfectly positioned to modulate the speed, amplitude and likelihood of motor movements. The neurodegenerative loss of this substantia nigra-striatum connection and the loss of the modulatory dopamine influence is responsible for most of the visible symptoms of Parkinson's disease. Without this dopamine modulation in the striatum, slowness, impaired walking, stiffness or tremor ensue.

The neurodegenerative loss of the substantia nigra and its dopamine modulation of the striatum was recognized years ago to be the substrate for most of the Parkinson's disease (PD) symptoms. This became the basis for PD treatment, i.e., replenishment of brain dopamine. Oral (and intravenous) dopamine cannot enter the brain and dopamine pills can provide no benefit for people with Parkinson's disease. However, it was recognized in the 1960's that the immediate natural precursor of dopamine, levodopa (l-dopa) is transported into the brain and is easily converted into dopamine.

Levodopa administration proved to markedly improve Parkinson's disease symptoms but the response when this was first introduced was compromised by nausea and vomiting plus the need for very high doses. Scientists quickly appreciated that the problem related to the immediate conversion of levodopa to dopamine in the circulation, prior to brain entry. The enzyme that converts levodopa to dopamine is ubiquitous and present in the circulation (dopa decarboxylase). The solution was to design a molecule that would block that enzyme but not enter the brain. The solution was carbidopa, which cannot enter the brain but blocks the enzyme that converts levodopa to dopamine. (In other countries benserazide serves the same purpose as carbidopa). Hence, the standard of Parkinson's disease treatment became and remains carbidopa/levodopa.

Carbidopa/levodopa remains the best medication for treating Parkinson's disease and is responsible for the extension of PD longevity to near normality. However, dopamine is not the entire story and other symptoms occur early and late and do not have a dopamine basis.

Parkinson's disease (PD) tends to be a decades-long process starting with subtle and non-disabling symptoms, often predating by years the visible, classic PD movement symptoms (gait, tremor, stiffness and slowness). This precursor state is variably characterized by dream enactment behavior (REM sleep behavior), constipation, anxiety or smell loss, which may span up to 20 years and occasionally longer.

These very early symptoms do not reflect loss of brain dopamine. The recognizable Parkinson's disease state with visible tremor, slowness, etc., represents an intermediate stage characterized by loss of the substantia nigra and the inherent dopamine. In this scenario, this represents the second and third stages of Parkinson's disease.

Note that the loss of the substantia nigra neurons responsible for the tremor, stiffness and walking problems is slow and visible symptoms are not apparent until dopamine neuron depletion reaches perhaps 50-60%. Estimates suggest that the dopamine neuron loss begins around 5-6 years before the movement symptoms become apparent.

The evolution of Parkinson's disease obviously does not end with the appearance of PD symptoms. What might be regarded as the 3rd PD stage reflects the ongoing slow additional loss of the dopamine system (dopaminergic substantia nigra). Over several years, the progressive loss of dopamine-containing substantia nigra neurons results in instability of the levodopa treatment response. At that point, there are not enough surviving substantia nigra nerve terminals to maintain a stable level of dopamine at their connection with the striatum. One might speculate that this may occur when the substantia nigra depletion is on the order of 10-20% of baseline. At that juncture, the medication, levodopa (carbidopa levodopa), generates less consistent responses, plus with changing response dynamics. Specifically, this is when people with Parkinson's disease develop the so-called, "wearing-off" responses and sometimes with involuntary movements called "dyskinesia". These are treatable by way of medication adjustments but symptom control is often imperfect. This 3rd stage tends to persist for a number of years.

As this third stage continues, the Parkinson's disease neurodegenerative process slowly starts to extend beyond the dopamine circuits. In other words, brain regions are affected where dopamine is not the signaling neurotransmitter and dopamine replenishment for these accompanying symptoms provides no benefit. Hence, after years in the third stage, the movement response to carbidopa/levodopa becomes less complete (still beneficial but less so than early in the course). .

Through these first 3 stages of Parkinson's disease, people with PD typically do reasonably well and often do not require much help with activities of daily living. To variable degrees, however, people with long-standing Parkinson's disease may start to reduce certain activities. At this point, family or spouses may need to take on more of the maintenance of the household. Many tasks and activities that were taken for granted in years past may need to be scaled back, such as landscaping projects or major household repairs. .Also, with more complex medication regimens the spouse or other family members may prove helpful by interceding with the clinician or provide insight about the dosage and timing of medications. However, through these three stages, people with Parkinson's disease usually do reasonably well.

Not to be forgotten is involvement of the autonomic nervous system, which may become more problematic with passing years of Parkinson's disease. The autonomic nervous system is responsible for bladder, bowel and blood pressure regulation. Symptoms that may develop include urinary urgency or incontinence, constipation or low blood pressure when standing.

The fourth PD stage is marked by the PD neurodegenerative process extending well beyond the dopamine motor system and especially affecting non-dopamine brain regions responsible for cognition, as well as movement control. Carbidopa/levodopa will still be necessary but the movement responses will be less complete; cognitive and autonomic symptoms will not benefit from this medication. Some with Parkinson's disease pass through this final stage without much upheaval beyond the effects of aging; however, for many, a kind, compassionate and dedicated caregiver is a real blessing.

To summarize, the advanced stages of Parkinson's disease may be experienced by an incomplete levodopa effect and cognitive impairment. For many, caregiving is of crucial importance. That is the special focus of this book, beautifully written by Dr. Klos.

J. Eric Ahlskog, Ph.D., M.D.

Professor of Neurology

Mayo Clinic, Rochester, MN

INTRODUCTION

Gerald was a typical fourteen-year-old boy, growing up in the Midwest. For quite a long time he had been saving credits at a local department store, which could be redeemed for merchandise. He knew what he wanted – A new bicycle. He had his eye on exactly the bike he wanted. He had been saving these store credits for what seemed like eternity. Now he was about to reach his target and excitedly told his father that he was reaching his goal and getting a new bike. His father was happy for him; they were a middle-class family and money was tight and too tight at that time to buy a bicycle.

When his father was at work later that week, a friend and co-worker mentioned that his daughter's birthday was coming up soon but he had not saved enough money to buy her the birthday present that she really wanted. Ironically, she also had her eye on a new bicycle. Her father's friend loved his daughter very much and felt bad that he could not come up with the money.

That evening when Gerald's father came home, he told Gerald about his friend's daughter and her wish for a birthday bicycle. Gerald didn't say much but could not stop thinking about this. Later that night, he found his father in the living room and told him that he wanted to give the store credits to his father's friend to buy his daughter the bike. Gerald's father asked him if he was certain he wanted to do this; after all, he had also been hoping for a new bike for a long time. Gerald had already made up his mind and this made his father very proud of him. The next day, the transaction was completed; his father gave Gerald's store credits to his co-worker and his daughter received the beautiful new bicycle she had been hoping for.

Gerald is now a grown man; actually a senior citizen. He told me this story one day in the clinic. Life took a funny turn several years after giving up his bicycle. He met the girl who had gotten the bicycle and ultimately fell in love with her. The love was mutual and they married. With a twinkle in his eyes as he stared at his wife with Parkinson's disease (PD) sitting in the wheelchair three feet away, he said, "She didn't know until the day we were married that I was the one who gave her the store credits for that bicycle she always wanted. I have been taking care of her ever since that day, fifty-eight years of marriage, and eighteen years as her caregiver for Parkinson's disease. It was meant to be that I would be caring for her and I wouldn't trade the honor and privilege of being her partner for anything!"

Are you a caregiver for a loved one with Parkinson's disease (PD)? If so, I can relate. I am a Neurologist, specializing in Movement Disorders. I take care of thousands of Parkinson patients and their caregivers in my clinical practice but I am also a caregiver to my mother who battles PD. I join millions of caregivers across the globe who aim to do the best job they possibly can to take care of, support, and love a family member with PD.

It is easy to develop a negative disposition about having to now care for someone with a chronic illness. Some individuals even leave their partner with PD because the journey of a caregiver is too scary and frankly not a journey the spouse is willing to take. The difficult choice is to opt-out or to be ready to serve our loved one with PD. I want you to join me in approaching PD caregiving with a servant attitude.

CONDUCTING THE RESEARCH FOR THIS BOOK

To learn more about the experience of Parkinson's disease caregivers and how they are handling different situations, I decided to research the topic in great detail with the caregivers in my practice. We interviewed two hundred and fifty willing caregivers and asked them to complete exhaustive questionnaires on numerous issues. The participants completed these interviews and questionnaires in confidence, away from the patient. Caregivers remained anonymous in reporting their thoughts, feelings, concerns, and advice to us.

The caregivers who participated in this project were a diverse group encompassing spouses, parents, children, siblings, relatives, and friends of the patient. These caregivers ranged in age from young adults to elderly individuals and lived in a variety of settings, including major cities, small towns, rural communities, and everywhere in between. A minority of the caregivers we interviewed now live apart from their loved one as the patient was moved into a nursing home facility or a memory care center. However, these individuals still spend the majority of their day at the living center at the side of the patient. They are still in the middle of the action in the day-to-day care of their loved one.

The majority of the care-giving spouses were retired; however, some caregivers worked outside the home. Some of these caregivers went back to work after becoming a caregiver for their loved one to meet the financial obligations of the family. The caregivers were from diverse racial and ethnic backgrounds. They participated in a variety of religions, and some had quit practicing their faith tradition. Most of the caregivers had completed at least a high school degree.

Some of the caregivers were financially stable, while others were living on a fixed income with great concern over their finances. A caregiver recently told me, "I don't know how we can continue to afford her medications. The cost of her care is emptying out the bank account. We never thought of buying long term care insurance when we were younger. This retirement money that was earmarked for us in the golden years to travel and enjoy retirement is dwindling away."

Caregivers varied in their own health status. Some of the caregivers were in excellent health and could take on the caregiving duties with great resolve and strength. Many people, however, were struggling to keep up with the requirements of caring for someone with PD.

Caregivers can be frail from the effects of aging and/or medical illness. They may not be able to lift a fallen loved one. One of our caregivers who provided excellent support for this project over the years passed away recently from a lung condition, leaving his loved one with PD alone in a nursing home. His greatest fear over the years was dying before she did. He spent all those years worrying about something over which he had no control. Despite his worries, he could not change the future.

In this book I outline the principles of caregiving that these care partners and patients shared with my team. With this information I hope it helps you rethink your role as a care partner or caregiver and build confidence and pride in the hard work yet fulfilling work you are facing.

WHAT MAKES THIS BOOK DIFFERENT?

In addition to my experience and feedback from caregivers and patients over the years, I have personal experience as a PD caregiver for my mom. My insight into the challenges that caregivers face deepened as I moved from being solely a medical professional to a medical professional *and* a caregiver. As I watch the disease progress in her I continue to learn more about the complexity of the various issues experienced by PD caregivers. This rare and unique perspective emerges from a practice full of PD patients and caregivers.

In the clinic many caregivers would ask me questions like, "What is the right way to deal with this situation?" or "How do I make the right choice in deciding to keep my loved one at home or move the patient into a living facility?" There are so many different approaches and treatments available, and thus, one solution does not work for all patients and caregivers. I tell them to stop asking what the right way to give care is and instead ask which solution will work the best for their particularly unique situation.

Caregivers for Parkinson patients are unique. Each situation and each patient are different. Caregivers come from diverse backgrounds, demographics, and financial circumstances. Caregivers need to realize that there is no one right way of caring for a PD patient. You are the one responsible for providing care for your loved one, and therefore, whatever is working for your family and the patient is the right way to care. You have the most knowledge of your loved one and their needs, and therefore, your decisions and loving care are what is best for your patient.

This book is full of the wisdom that caregivers shared with us in our research project. You will find valuable insight into the world of caregiving for people with Parkinson. They taught us many lessons they have learned over the years while performing one of the most challenging jobs on the planet: Caregiving. I hope that what they have learned is helpful for you.

CHAPTER 1

CARE PARTNER IN EARLY-STAGE PARKINSON'S DISEASE

CARE PARTNER IN EARLY-STAGE PARKINSON'S DISEASE

Many people with PD and their care partners have realized that PD was already causing symptoms well before they were given the actual diagnosis. During the years that they experienced these symptoms, they were unaware as to the relationship with early PD. It was not until they were educated on the research of preclinical PD that a connection was clear.

For example, I was interviewing a patient named Fred who was accompanied by his wife. I asked Fred if he had experienced a change in bowel habits over the recent years. Fred admitted that his bowels had always been regular until about six years ago when he developed the insidious onset of constipation. He never mentioned this to his primary doctor. Instead, he battled this problem with over the counter remedies, which worked reasonably well for him. When I asked Fred if he had noticed a change in his ability to smell or taste, he couldn't believe that he was answering yes to yet another question of past symptoms. Fred told me that he thought it was odd that he lost so much recognition of common smells like the beautiful aroma of his morning coffee.

I asked Fred about symptoms of anxiety or depression. Fred did not immediately admit to a history of emotional changes. However, his wife quickly jumped in and told me, "Yes! Fred has become so anxious. He worries about everything, which is not like him. We rarely go out to new places or try unfamiliar plans with friends because he has a hard time handling these situations."

Experts in the field of PD have recognized that a group of preclinical symptoms may develop in individuals for at least five to six years or more before they are diagnosed with PD. Four common changes may develop for people with PD including anxiety, loss of smell, constipation, and REM sleep behavior disorder. REM sleep behavior disorder is a nighttime behavior in which the individual acts out their dream typically manifested by kicking, jerking, fighting, or other involuntary movements. Normally, when we dream, our body remains still as we sleep. However, with REM sleep behavior disorder the brain no longer inhibits the motor system; thus, allowing the body to move as ordered by the dream.

Another care partner named Theresa gave me an excellent description of this behavior. Theresa described her husband's behavior to me. She said, "My husband is a policeman here in our town. I thought he was just becoming more and more stressed at work. During the night, I would wake up to a loud scream or sometime shouting from my husband. I looked over at him and he was screaming out in his sleep. I couldn't believe the words he was saying; he was obviously upset with someone. Then he started to swing in the air above him as if he was trying to beat someone up. I quickly moved away from him and thankfully missed a few punches coming my way. He eventually grabbed his pillow and put the pillow in a choke hold like I had never seen. He caught the bad guy he was after, no doubt. I'm just thankful it wasn't me that he grabbed like that!"

Theresa later learned all about REM sleep behavior disorder. Thankfully, this behavior did not occur nightly but often enough to alarm her. Eventually, one night during one of his

REM sleep behavior outbursts, her husband flung himself out of bed during a dream and hit his head on the night table. On that occasion, they ended up traveling to the emergency room where he received ten sutures across the forehead to mend the laceration.

PD researchers have learned that the pathological process of PD may start more than even twenty years before the patient is diagnosed. Over these years prior to diagnosis, PD patients may experience these pre-clinical symptoms of anxiety, REM sleep behavior disorder, constipation, and diminished smell. Pathologists have discovered that the pathological changes of PD are in the body and are found in locations that correlate with these early symptoms. The spread of PD pathology continues slowly over the years until it reaches the upper brainstem region of the brain at which time the classic motor symptoms of PD result. These motor symptoms include tremor, slowness of movement (bradykinesia), and stiffness or rigidity of limb movements.

When I explained preclinical PD to Fred and his wife, they were shocked to learn that even though his tremor, slow movement, and stiff arm and leg had just developed within the last three months, that PD was already in his brain for many years and he had no idea. He now realized that the symptoms of constipation and anxiety were due to the disease. All of these changes that Fred had experienced were now coming together into a new understanding.

Over time, these pathological changes of PD found in the brain may continue to spread. Fortunately, for most people, this spread is very slow and may span decades of time. My mom is a good example of this. She had experienced an increase in anxiety and change in smell for many years. Then when she developed a tremor in her hands, it seemed to me and her doctors that she was just dealing with an isolated tremor condition such as Essential tremor. She had no other motor signs for several years. Her gait was normal and her speed of movement seemed to be appropriate for her age. In retrospect, we may not have realized how much her movement was slowing down. There were simply not enough symptoms to arrive at a diagnosis of Parkinson's disease until one day she stumbled at home walking from one room to the next. She told me her feet were shuffling a bit and she had trouble picking them up and caught the rug with her toes. Eventually, the slowing down of her movements, the gait changes, and the tremor led us to the diagnosis of PD.

When I told her that I suspected that she may be dealing with early PD, she didn't believe me.

I said, "Mom, this is my specialty of practice. I am an expert in PD. Why don't you believe me?"

She said, "Oh, I just don't believe I have that condition. I just have a tremor and I am getting older. You know I have a degenerative lumbar spine so I probably just tripped due to my back."

To settle the disagreement, I ordered a brain scan called a DAT scan. This is a type of a nuclear imaging test of the brain that allows the radiologist to determine if an individual has a deficit in dopamine. This deficit of dopamine is diagnostic for conditions like Parkinson's disease and allows us to differentiate Parkinson's disease from Essential tremor. Her scan came back positive for PD and she eventually accepted the diagnosis.

YOU AS A CARE PARTNER

It may seem odd discussing caregiving in the early stages of PD since most patients in the early stages are fully independent. These early stages may involve up to ten to fifteen years after diagnosis or sometimes even longer. If the patient is over the age of eighty, then the duration of early stage PD may be substantially shorter.

Most patients who are started on medication may not show any visible signs of PD. Many of my early-stage PD patients boast to me that, "No one can tell I even have PD." This, of course, helps the patient maintain employment and pursue hobbies as if nothing has really changed. At this stage, you are really a care partner and not a caregiver.

People with early stage PD have mostly a "normal" appearance. However, the diagnosis brings forth a level of anxiety and concern for all involved. There are abundant fears about the future. What will this condition bring to my loved one? How will our lives change? What kind of help will we need? There are so many questions clouding our minds at this stage.

Intermixed with the questions of concern about the future is a feeling of relief for most care partners in that a diagnosis has been issued. Many patients go months or years before the diagnosis is made. Patients may have had many different health care provider visits, visits to specialists, and many tests run before arriving at the diagnosis. The fear of the unknown may become overwhelming. Now that we know what illness we are facing, we are relieved to hear that treatments are available.

Care partners find great comfort in seeing their loved one improve as health providers prescribe medication for their PD. Tremors may subside or even abate. The shuffling walk slowly improves and the patient reports less discomfort from the slowness and stiffness. The patient's muscle pain may have improved.

If we look at the longitudinal perspective of how PD progresses, many people are pleasantly surprised that the forecast is not as grim as they thought. When patients are diagnosed and started on treatment, they will typically go on to do quite well for the next ten to fifteen years. Over these years, there is the opportunity to continue working if the individual is employed or wishes to work. Many retirees will take advantage of their retirement years and travel around the country or abroad. Some will pick up new hobbies or volunteer work and be able to stay in the mainstream of life.

It is during these early years that PD results in primarily a dopamine deficiency state within the brain and the dopamine replacement medication replenishes dopamine to the brain. It is not until the later stages, perhaps ten or more years later, that more problems may surface due to the spread of PD into other brain regions. When this happens a variety of new problems may present involving non-dopamine motor pathways, cognitive and visuospatial networks, and other automatic regulatory circuits of the brain that modulate blood pressure, heart rate responses, bowel and bladder function, and sweating ability for example.

During the first decade or longer, the spouse or family member is best described as a care partner. The patient remains independent but they do need love and support as well as to have someone to accompany them to medical appointments as needed. The role of the care partner is mostly to be an advocate for their loved one and to be aware of what is happening with the patient as well as in the medical world that may help their loved one.

I find that most spouses or family members that witness the official rendering of the diagnosis may not truly understand what is to be expected in the years to come and often have a much more pessimistic outlook on the future. Many care partners felt confused about how much to help their loved one with certain daily tasks versus being patient while the patient attempts to perform the task independently. For example, a care partner observed their loved one with PD taking over thirty minutes to chop up one vegetable for a meal that they were cooking together. The person with PD became irritated when the care partner tried to take over the job of cutting for them because they wanted to show that they were still capable of completing this task. The care partner wanted to help because they were losing patience.

As we surveyed care partners the most significant concern was in trying to understand what the future will be like for both their loved one and themselves. Their fears about the future really divided into two categories. The first category was concern about the patient and the second category was concern about their own future.

THE PHYSICAL CHANGES OF PARKINSON'S DISEASE

Care partners listed concerns about the physical and mental state of the patient as the disease advances. At the top of the list is the concern about the potential loss of mobility for the patient. Would their loved one be able to walk throughout the rest of their life, or will they require a wheelchair and full assistance to move? If they need a wheelchair, how much help will the loved one be able to give in transfers? How much lifting will be required to get them where they need to go? Will they be able to use a walker instead of being confined to a wheelchair?

Most patients in the early stages of PD need very little assistance with their mobility and coordination, especially after starting symptomatic therapy. However, there is a progressive weakness that results and may cause difficulty with mobility later in the course if not addressed. Health care providers constantly stress to patients that they must exercise to keep their bodies as strong as possible and to keep themselves in a better position to fight the progression of the disease.

One of the challenges for the PD patient and the care partner is the commitment to exercise. Many patients were not athletes in their earlier years. Many patients have never had an interest in exercising before the PD diagnosis. Now the thought of going to the gym or exercise class seems as foreign an idea as living on Mars. Patients fight the battle of limited motivation to exercise coupled with motor challenges of PD. Compounding these challenges may result in some patients experiencing fatigue and variable levels of apathy.

Jim's Story

Jim admitted to me that the last time that he performed any meaningful exercise was twenty-five years ago when he used to work out at the YMCA. Due to demands at work and general laziness, he stopped working out over the years and now faced the onset of PD. For over a year, Jim ignored my advice to start an exercise program. It was now three years into the disease process from the time of diagnosis and close to five years since the first sign that PD had affected his body.

I sat with Jim and his family at one visit and listened to him describing the progressive weakness and muscle atrophy that he was noticing over the years. Jim knew how important exercise and muscle strength building is in treating PD. The problem was that he really did not know where to start, lacked the motivation to get started, and had no one to hold him accountable for his workouts. It was during that visit that his adult son, who lived only five miles from Jim, decided to intervene. I stressed how important exercise is to Jim and his family, and his son decided that he was not going to let his father slip away without a fight.

Jim's son decided to take an active role in his father's care. He told his father in the exam room that from now on, six days a week, he will be going with his father to the local gym and exercising together. Over the years, Jim and his son have rarely missed a workout together. His son helped him regain his comfort on the resistance machines three days a week and motivated him to slowly add more aerobic fitness on the treadmill, stationary bike, and other equipment. It was very important that his dopamine medication was optimized in order to give him the ability to move and workout with maximal efficiency.

Over the subsequent years, Jim's family and I witnessed significant improvement in his strength and mobility. The progressive decline was certainly slowed by their hard work. They added additional classes for PD, including a local boxing program. Jim and his son realized that having a workout partner to hold Jim accountable and keep him motivated was the key to success with exercise. Jim not only enjoyed the benefits of the exercise class but relished the time he spent with his son. Together their relationship grew closer and both realized how much love and support they could be for each other.

Exercise and strength are the next important issue. We now know that a key part of the treatment paradigm for PD is incorporating exercise from the very beginning and all the way through the advanced stages. The more the patient engages in resistance and strength-building activities, cardiovascular fitness, and stretching, the better they will do in the later stages.

This is an excellent opportunity for the care partner to step in and to actively help their loved one. We all maintain consistency in exercising when we have an accountability partner. If you are physically able as a care partner, step up and be their exercise partner. Help motivate each other to be consistent and faithful to the program. Both of you will benefit greatly!

CREATING AN EXERCISE PROGRAM

The first step is to assess what you, the care partner, may safely do in the form of exercise and what resources you have nearby. Check with your primary care provider and receive clearance for an exercise program appropriate for your age and your health condition. Next, make sure your loved one also has medical approval for an appropriate exercise program. Find out what the Neurologist recommends for exercise. There are many options available for PD patients and their care partners. Discover and commit to a program that both of you may enjoy.

If your loved one with PD already exercises regularly and independently of you, you may offer to be their accountability partner. Consider approaching this discussion in saying that you are committed to exercising too so let's help motivate each other and keep each other accountable. Be watchful to see if there is a progressive loss of motivation to keep up the schedule. If you are not exercising regularly, this is a great time to make changes in your life.

You will benefit greatly from the exercise. Exercise is a great way to reduce stress and to keep your body in optimal health. Furthermore, you will maintain your strength and health to be a better caregiver over the long term.

If you are a care partner who is limited in your ability to exercise or cannot participate in exercise, then you can still motivate and encourage your loved one to be consistent in their program. Be the driver to the boxing class, for example. Many of my caregivers have enjoyed going to the boxing class twice a week. While the PD patients are in the one hour class, working with the instructor, all of the care partners go into the lobby and have an impromptu caregiver support meeting. These care partners share ideas and their experiences with each other. They enjoy the camaraderie of others who understand what they are going through. This is a precious time for the care partners. Both the care partner and the patient benefit, and by going together they stay motivated to keep up the schedule.

In the early stages of PD the goal is to keep the patient's body strong and to keep them as active as possible. This means optimizing medication from the provider and optimizing the exercise program. Although every situation doesn't guarantee that the patient will always be independent in mobility and be able to live at home until their death, these programs greatly improve the likelihood of better outcomes.

Although a randomized, placebo-controlled, clinical trial has not been performed to date in PD related to exercise and the potential to slow progression, there are numerous, in fact hundreds of studies, reported in medical journals that would support using exercise in the treatment of PD. A great summary of the potential neuroprotective effects of exercise for PD may be found in *The New Parkinson's Disease Treatment* book, second edition, by Dr. JE Ahlskog or in his article – Ahlskog, JE., Does vigorous exercise have a neuroprotective effect in Parkinson's disease? Neurology 2011, 77:288-294.

The body of research indicates that we live longer and have better outcomes if we exercise aerobically on a regular basis. This means a type of exercise that maintains an elevated heart rate, causes us to perspire and breathe hard. There are so many options that may suit the ability of the individual and may address any medical or orthopedic challenges. For instance, if bad knees prevent a patient from running on a treadmill, then pedaling a recumbent stationary bike might be a better option. It is important that your loved one with PD receive medical clearance by their medical health care provider before engaging in aerobic exercise. After clearance, they should start slow and build up their endurance over time in a controlled fashion. Eventually, it is recommended to perform at least thirty minutes of moderate exercise at least five days a week or to perform vigorous-intensity aerobic workouts for at least twenty minutes on three days a week.

In order to maintain muscle strength, I recommend to my patients that resistance exercise such as pushing or pulling against an appropriate weight such as the weight machines at the local gym at least twice a week is advantageous. If free weights and/or machines are available in your home, this may be a reasonable substitute for a gym membership. If we let aging and PD continue to cause atrophy of muscles and weakness especially in the core muscles, then PD patients will be more prone to falls and have more difficulty with their mobility. This will put additional burdens on the care partner as you will need to provide more daily assistance for mobility.

There are cognitive and psychological benefits from exercise as well. Research has convincingly demonstrated that daily exercise is capable of lowering the risk of dementia. In addition, more recent research using MRI imaging of the brain has shown that aerobic exercise performed three days a week results in neurogenesis or an increase in brain volume within the hippocampus region of the brain, which is responsible for memory function. Psychiatrist have recognized that mood improves with exercise similar to what they observe from antidepressant medication trials. A study in the *Journal of Neurology* by a research group in Pittsburg showed that walking six to nine miles per week may help to preserve brain volume and mitigate the cognitive decline of aging seen in later life.

DOPAMINE REPLACEMENT THERAPY

I vividly remember the first time I evaluated a patient with Parkinson's disease in the clinic. I watched an elderly man sitting on the exam room couch as if frozen like a statue. His face appeared mask-like. He rarely blinked. His hands were frozen on his lap almost with a perfect 90 degree bend at the elbow. Both feet lay motionless on the floor. As I began the interview it took him several seconds to turn his head in my direction. It seemed like hours before he was able to respond to my questions and when he did, he responded in a soft whisper of a voice.

My patient revealed that he had not yet taken his first dose of dopamine medication that morning. He wanted me to see him while off his medication. I asked him to stand from the chair and walk in the hallway. After numerous attempts to rock back and forth, he finally used his arms to push his elderly body into the air where he stood with a stooped posture. He took several steps in place to turn and face the exam room door. Eventually he was able to slowly shuffle his way to the door.

When the exam was completed, I asked him to go ahead and take his dopamine medication. I told him that I would re-examine him in one hour when the medication had taken affect. He gladly swallowed his medication and waited patiently.

I returned to his exam room about an hour and a half later. Sitting back on the exam room chair was the same patient but at first I could not believe that this was the same man. He was spontaneously looking around the room with a gentle smile on his face. His eyes were blinking and he quickly responded faster to my questions with a much stronger voice. Now, he was able to stand up from the chair without using his arms and he did not require multiple attempts to stand. He pivoted in place and moved across the room and out the door. He walked up and down the hall with an almost normal posture and improved stride. This patient looked like a different man than the one I had left in the exam room over an hour ago. This type of response to the dopamine medication is typical for a PD patient.

In the early to mid 1900s, scientist made a revolutionary discovery related to dopamine. It was discovered that patients with Parkinson's disease have a fundamental and progressive loss of the brain neurochemical named dopamine. Scientists discovered a way to package the precursor to dopamine named levodopa into a pill. The pill could be swallowed and the levodopa would cross into the brain. Levodopa inside the brain is converted into dopamine by a brain enzyme and now dopamine is readily available to restore communication in motor pathways.

Dopamine is an important neurotransmitter in the brain responsible for communicating in the motor circuit. Without adequate dopamine, the brain fails to command muscles of our body to move automatically at the normal speed and amplitude. Thus, a patient with Parkinson's disease blinks infrequently, swallows less, and has less spontaneous movements. Hence, for example, we observe the mask-like face of a Parkinson disease patient.

Dopamine is vital for the execution of voluntary movements. When a patient with Parkinson's disease desires to stand up from the chair or perform simple tasks like writing or buttoning a shirt, the movements performed become slow and restricted in range of motion. The slow and restricted movements lead to a feeling of weakness for the patient. There are times when the brain commands a movement but the body does not respond. These episodes are referred to as freezing.

Paradoxically, 75 percent of patients with Parkinson's disease experience tremors from this deficiency of dopamine. A region of the brain creates a tremor signal, which rhythmically transmits an impulse four to six times per second out from the brain and out to the limbs of the body. Most commonly, the tremor is seen in the hand and/or arm muscles. However, the signal may transmit to the leg or even the chin. Some patients will experience the tremor on the inside of their body as if their internal organs are shaking. Dopamine replacement medication is also capable of treating the Parkinson's disease tremor. Once dopamine levels are restored in the brain, the tremor signal abates and both the internal and external shaking resolves.

PREPARING FOR THE MENTAL CHANGES OF
A PD PATIENT

A common concern from care partners regarding the future of the patient is the concern about how the patient will change mentally. In my clinic, nearly 50 percent of early PD patients experience mild cognitive changes independent of age. These changes seem to vary between short-term memory loss, executive dysfunction, and visuospatial changes. Care partners worry about dementia, specifically. What will happen when my loved one has trouble remembering day to day information? Will they remember me? Will they be able to take care of themselves or will I have to manage everything for them? Will I have to bathe them, change them, feed them?

The reality is that most PD patients will remain cognitively strong for many years and even more than a decade after the diagnosis. If a PD patient is still employed at the time of diagnosis, they may often continue working for many years without any difficulty. The dopamine medication prescribed helps the PD patient to be able to work and continue within the mainstream of life. If the PD patient is a retiree, they may certainly engage in the usual activities of retirement.

I continue to advise patients and care partners to meet with an attorney to establish essential safeguards in place for the future. First, it is crucial to set up an Advanced Directive. This legal document allows the patient to spell out specifically their wishes for care at the end of life to avoid confusion from family members and healthcare providers. Second, a durable Power of Attorney for healthcare is a document that should be created to officially name the family member who will be the patients' healthcare proxy. The proxy is the individual who will make healthcare decisions for the patient, if they are unable to do so. Third, many care partners and the patient have consulted with an Accountant to discuss financial planning and tax related information to plan for the future. It is never too early to start planning for the future.

I believe it is also imperative to discuss as a couple or family the approach to driving. Driving is a potentially dangerous activity for patients with PD as the disease advances. Not only their life is at stake but also innocent people on the road. It is essential to work closely as a team with the health care providers in determining the safety of driving. I also recommend that patients go to the motor vehicle department at least every six months and receive a formal driving test with their staff. If the department deems the patient safe to operate a vehicle, then you can alleviate a lot of concerns every six months. This approach reduces potential conflict between you and the patient should the time come when the patient needs to surrender driving privileges. If the patient is unable to pass a driving test by the motor vehicle department, then they should not be driving, and the motor vehicle department will take the privilege away so that you are not the bad guy.

MOM'S DRIVING

Early in the course of the illness, I knew my mom was already noticing some mild cognitive changes in visuospatial skills. The first problem was her calling me to tell me that she backed the car out of the garage down the driveway and ran over the metal mailbox located in the grass near the driveway. I dismissed this event as just an accident and thought this could happen to anyone. I was happy to replace her mailbox and move on. Shortly after that episode, she told me she parked too close to another car in the shopping center and scratched the side of their car. Next, she backed out of a parking spot and hit a concrete pole denting in part of her bumper. I noticed on another occasion when she parked next to my vehicle that she had failed to pull all the way into the parking stall and left about four feet of space in front of the car. The visuospatial cognitive changes are one of the PD related changes that may lead to the loss of driving privileges.

In addition to cognitive concerns is the concern of the patient's psychological changes. Now that television commercial ads are playing about PD psychosis, highlighting the visual hallucinations and delusional thoughts that patients may experience, care partners are naturally fearful of the future. The commercial is alarming suggesting that PD patients will commonly experience these problems. In my practice, psychosis is not a common problem for patients. If hallucinations or confusion become a new symptom for a patient, the majority of these patients will respond to a medication capable of resolving this psychosis.

Care partners are also concerned about depression and anxiety symptoms. They ask, "What will I do if my loved one is so depressed that they don't want to do anything but just stay in bed all day?" "What do I do if they are so anxious that they won't leave the house to be with other people?" "How will I get them to exercise if they refuse to be active and leave the house?"

"What if our relationship changes because the patient is depressed and less social, more irritated, and at times difficult to be around? How will I handle this?"

In our survey of caregivers, the respondents identified anxiety about PD's psychological changes as a significant concern. Early on, many care partners may already be aware of the changes in emotions. They may observe depression symptoms in their loved one. They may see their loved one's anxiety levels increasing. It is very unlikely for the care partner to observe psychotic symptoms.

If psychotic symptoms develop, tell your health care provider right away as an immediate work-up is necessary and more than likely the psychotic symptoms are resulting from some other cause. This may be a treatable cause such as a urinary tract infection.

TRANSFERRING RESPONSIBILITY FOR FINANCIAL MANAGEMENT

Patients may struggle with keeping the checkbook balanced. If the patient is the one who prepares the family taxes, then changes may need to be implemented. It is essential for the care partner to monitor the payment of bills, balancing the checkbook, making financial decisions and preparing taxes. As a care partner, we want the patient to remain independent as long as possible in doing the usual daily tasks of the family. However, patients are now at a higher risk of making mistakes due to the mild cognitive changes of PD; thus, the family needs to be guarded against such errors.

A patient of mine years ago always handled the family taxes. A few years after the diagnosis of PD, the patient could not mentally figure out the correct way to prepare the tax report. His wife had never been a part of the process, so she assumed he knew what he was doing and assumed that her husband would tell someone if he needed help or could no longer do the taxes independently. Unfortunately, this patient did not recognize his errors and continued to submit the tax forms each year with major errors. Eventually, the IRS audited the family and he was found guilty of hundreds of thousands of dollars of tax violations. The care partner was caught entirely off guard and asked me to write a letter to the IRS explaining that he was not mentally competent. Over the years, he was mentally competent to make decisions but unfortunately, the mild cognitive changes prevented him from correctly calculating and reporting the tax information properly on the form.

Another concern at this stage for care partners relates to future finances. Care partners and their families ask, "Will our family have the financial resources to pay for the care needed?"

"What does our long-term care policy cover if we even have one?" Some care partners recognize that the patient is involved in a family business, which may have an unknown future. "Will the company continue to run with the loved one still involved? Or will we need to sell the business and if so, when?" "What kind of income will we have to survive?" "Will I have to go to work or continue to work to support our family? If so, who will take care of my loved one while I work?"

"If I am an adult child of the patient, how will I balance my work obligations, immediate family needs, and caregiving for my parent?" These are important questions to resolve in the early years. Meeting with a Financial Planner and a Disability Attorney may be a crucial first step to giving both of you peace of mind and creating a financial strategy to follow as the disease progresses.

PERSONAL CONCERNS

Care partners have concerns about their own future. Most care partners worry about whether they will have the ability to care for their loved ones in the future when their loved one is in the most need of their help. Care partners are concerned that if they are not able to care for their loved one, then who will take care of their loved one, and will that person or persons be capable of caring for the loved one like the care partner would care for them? This is especially true if there is no other family member capable of providing care; thus, if the care partner was not around, then the patient would have to live in a nursing home. Care partners are anxious about that idea. They lament over whether nursing home staff will treat the loved one well and take care of them when the loved one is most vulnerable.

Unfortunately, considerable variability exists in the quality of the nursing home centers and staff. In most nursing home facilities, staff shortages create a poverty of proper care for the residents. Patients and caregivers tell me frequently of the horror stories they hear about the type of care some PD patients have received in certain facilities. There are many good care facilities and some with even additional training in the care of PD patients. Consulting with local PD support groups or agencies may direct you to the best facilities to consider should the need arise.

Next, care partners raise the concern that they may not be supportive enough to their loved one now or in the future. They fear that they are not listening enough to the patient's concerns. The care partner may think they need to solve all problems and take care of any concerns. Sometimes patients don't need a fix immediately but just want someone to listen to them. They want to be heard and to know that their caregiver is giving them loving concern and empathy. It is often therapeutic for people, especially with a chronic illness like PD, to be able to verbalize their feelings and symptoms to let someone else know what they are going through. It helps to feel validated that their symptoms are real, serious, and due to their illness.

Care partners are often busy and in a rush. Thus, they don't always have the luxury of being able to sit patiently and listen. Of course, listening to the patient and not reacting to try to fix everything might be precisely what the patient needs to feel better. Care partners worry that they are failing to listen and support their loved ones enough. They worry about rushing the patient to complete tasks and to finish their sentences. In many situations, the care partner may jump in and talk for the patient to prevent others from waiting on the patient to finish their thoughts. This may at times undermine the dignity of the patient. Often, the patient will withdraw from conversations and just let the family member do all the talking rather than participate in the conversations.

In my practice, I encourage care partners to always be patient with their loved ones. Give them time to complete sentences, and allow plenty of time to complete motor tasks such as eating or dressing. If the patient just cannot complete the task, then let them ask for assistance. There are some situations where the care partner might have to jump in right away with assistance so that they are not late for an appointment for example.

PROGNOSIS OF PARKINSON'S DISEASE (PD)

The life expectancy of a person with PD is nearly that of the general population. PD results in only a relatively small life span reduction overall. The main reason for such longevity with a neurodegenerative disorder is the introduction of dopamine replacement therapy, which was introduced in the US market around 1969 to 1970. This dopamine medication, levodopa, restores the brain neurotransmitter, dopamine, and allows individuals with PD to improve their mobility, strength, motor function and ultimately their lifespan.

The long-term course may be complicated by several factors. First, an aging brain will have an additive affect on PD symptoms especially related to cognition, motor skills, and balance. We have observed in our neurology practice that consistently when individuals reach the age of eighty, aging causes an apparent change in balance. Over time, seniors over eighty years of age need to adapt to this balance change by moving slower, avoiding ladders or other potentially dangerous equipment, and being extra careful when bending over to pick up objects from the floor.

In addition to aging, patients may have a variety of different orthopedic and/or spine disorders that may affect mobility and balance. For example, a degenerative knee condition may affect a patients ability to stand up from the chair. A cane or walker may be necessary to prevent the knee from giving way and causing a fall. Medications may have side effects that affect the nervous system. Blood pressure medications for example may cause PD patients to have low blood pressure episodes that cause dizziness, lightheadedness, weakness and even at times syncope (black-outs). The older one is with PD, the likelihood of an individual experiencing cardiovascular problems and/or strokes also complicate the prognosis of PD.

There are other problems that may develop along the course including dementia. In our clinic, less than 40 percent of patients with PD develop dementia from PD. We have several medications currently available that might provide modest improvement in memory and thinking capabilities. The brains ability to regulate bowel and bladder function and blood pressure control may become problematic. During the first five to ten years, PD has minimal effect on these automatic functions of the nervous system but later a patient may experience more difficulties.

Overall, prognosis is difficult to predict. Each individual with PD will progress at variable rates. Age and other medical illnesses will affect the prognosis. Thankfully, PD tends to move slowly over decades for most individuals allowing for many good years together with your loved one.

CHAPTER 2

PARKINSON'S DISEASE IS TREATABLE

Sally's Story

Sally is a patient in our clinic who exemplifies the miraculous like effect of dopamine on her tremor. I will never forget watching her shake in the exam room chair. Sally had suffered with tremor for three years. Her whole body would shake rhythmically while at rest. The shaking also persisted with posture and movements of the limbs. She could not sip a drink out of a cup without spilling on herself or use a utensil without spilling the food.

I remember asking her to take a dose of carbidopa/levodopa in the office. About an hour later, I was amazed to find her sitting in the chair perfectly calm without any visible sign of tremor. What a miraculous treatment!

LEVODOPA THERAPY

When levodopa therapy was brought onto the market by 1970, it revolutionized the treatment of PD. Levodopa is the precursor molecule that is converted to dopamine inside the brain. By taking levodopa in the pill form, a patient replenishes the deficient neurotransmitter within the brain, which helps to restore motor function. Most, if not all, of the motor symptoms of PD will improve with this medication. The younger a patient using the medication, the better the response. With the improvement in mobility and muscle strength individuals with PD will live a longer lifespan and ultimately have a better quality of life.

Levodopa is the primary medication for Parkinson's disease patients. It is the most effective treatment available, and it is sold under the generic name of carbidopa/levodopa or the brand name of Sinemet. This medication is taken orally in the form of a tablet. After taking this medication, patients wait on average no more than an hour for the medication to work.

Early on in the disease process, there are still at least 50 percent of the dopamine neurons functioning properly. Thus, when the patient takes a dose of levodopa, it has a long and stable effect on the brain. Patients may find that if their timing of medicine is off an hour or two, they may not be able to tell a difference. The surviving dopamine neurons are still producing enough dopamine to compensate. In addition, neighboring brain cells are assisting the dopamine neurons as well. As the disease progresses and more dopamine neurons degenerate less natural dopamine is available; thus, the dopamine signaling capabilities are not as efficient as in the past. Now the patient is increasingly more dependent on the dopamine replacement and its timing taken by pill form.

As the dopamine neurons degenerate slowly over time the compensating brain cells are less efficient in properly signaling the dopamine receptors with the dopamine neurotransmitter. At times, excessive stimulation of the dopamine receptor may occur. The excessive stimulation leads to excessive involuntary movements. These movements are wiggling, chaotic, dance like movements of the body that can range from subtle to marked movements. The medical term for these movements is "dyskinesia." Most of my care partners understand what the movement looks like when I mention the movements they witness from Michael J. Fox when he is interviewed on TV. The younger the patient, the higher the risk of dyskinesia.

Another complication that may develop from the progressive deterioration of dopamine neurons is a problem called motor fluctuations. In this situation, the levodopa medication was taken for example in the morning after waking up from a night sleep. Usually, the patient could take the next dose of levodopa about six hours later. However, now they notice that after five hours, the benefit of the levodopa pill is fading quickly and they experience a return of PD symptoms during the hour before the next dose of medication was due. This is called "wearing off" of the dopamine response. The healthcare provider will troubleshoot this problem typically by recommending that the patient move the next dose earlier in the day by about an hour.

Through decades of experience and numerous studies, we have learned that a patient cannot save a better dopamine response for later in the course of the illness. Use of the medication earlier in the course will have no effect on the development of the complications of wearing off or dyskinesia. Thus, it is to the patient's advantage to use levodopa early after diagnosis and to use an adequate amount to control symptoms. Levodopa will continue working for the patient to the very end of their life. The duration of time that each pill lasts may change over time. Adjustments to the medication will be required and supplementary medications may be required as well. Some patients may require more advanced technologies such as deep brain stimulation or pump devices to treat these complications.

Levodopa has not been found to have any toxic effects on the brain or other bodily organs. No blood monitoring is required. Levodopa is the most effective treatment for PD, one that all patients will require. Some patients and healthcare providers may become concerned about using the treatment too early but studies and experience have informed us that there is no advantage to delaying levodopa therapy for later in the course.

LEVODOPA DOSING

It is important for care partners to understand how this medication works and how it is dosed so that you can better assist your love one.

First, it is important to know that levodopa is not given by itself. If an individual took a pill of pure levodopa then they would likely become ill with nausea and/or vomiting. Scientists discovered that if a medication named carbidopa was added to the pill of levodopa, then in most cases the nausea would be prevented. Occasionally, we may prescribe additional carbidopa if a patient still experiences nausea but this is quite rare.

The combination of carbidopa/levodopa has become the central and most important therapy for PD. The brand name is called Sinemet. In certain European countries and other countries outside of the US, a drug named benserazide replaces carbidopa and the combination has the brand name Madopar. These two medications are essentially interchangeable.

Carbidopa/levodopa works best if taken on an empty stomach in the absence of dietary protein. If a patient ingests a meal or snack consisting of protein (such as a hamburger and a milk shake), then a good portion of the carbidopa/levodopa medication will be blocked from entering the brain. Thus, I recommend taking the medication either at least an hour before a protein meal or snack or at least two hours after. This will allow for a consistent and full dose of carbidopa/levodopa to be absorbed into the brain. Please do not conclude that protein should be eliminated from the patient's diet. It is simply just important to pay attention to the timing of the carbidopa/levodopa medication and the ingestion of substantial protein in the food or drink.

The standard approach is to use the immediate release formulation of carbidopa/levodopa tablets. I recommend the 25/100 mg tablets as opposed to the 10/100 mg tablets so that the patient receives adequate dosing of carbidopa and therefore has the best chance of blocking nausea. The tablets are scored so that an incremental change of half a tablet may be used to titrate the medication to best result. I start patients off with one tablet taken three times a day, typically one hour before each of the three meals. If the patient does not eat three square meals a day, then we typically dose the medication every four to six hours while awake for the three doses.

After the first week of taking one tablet of carbidopa/levodopa three times a day, the patient may increase the medication by half a tablet each week to a maximum of three tablets per dose. The dose is raised each week until the optimal benefit is achieved without side effect. Once the optimal dose is found, the patient may continue on that dose. For example, if a patient reports that on week 3 of the medication titration process that the dose of two tablets taken three times a day is working very well to control symptoms without side effects, then the patient may remain on that dose. If the patient had tried taking two and a half tablets and found no additional benefit, then we recommend to the patient to take the lower of the two strengths. If side effects are experienced at any point along the titration process, then the patient will reduce the dose back to the previous dosing level.

Once carbidopa/levodopa therapy is optimized, other adjuvant PD medication is rarely necessary. With levodopa monotherapy a patient will have a lower risk of side effects and better response compared to the other PD medication options.

You can help your loved one with the timing of the medication. Find a schedule that works for your loved one and anchor the times of the medication consistently each day. Try to have a starting dose each morning taken at the same time so that the rest of the doses of the day can be taken at consistent times. This will allow for less chance of a forgotten dose or a delayed dose. You can help your loved one to be aware of potential conflicts with protein in the meals and snacks timed too close to the medication. You have the opportunity to help coordinate the meal times around the dosing times and not force the patient to dose the medication at a suboptimal time. Maintaining the proper dosing schedule will greatly reduce the chances of breakthrough symptoms of PD and minimize discomfort for the patient.

Over time the duration of benefit of the immediate release carbidopa/levodopa may shorten. Thus, the health care provider may ask the patient to take doses closer together to avoid the wearing off effect. There is no arbitrary limit to how many doses may be taken over a twenty-four hour period as long as side effects are not experienced. Typically, the strength of each dose does not need to be changed over time but just the number of doses taken per day.

WHICH FORM OF CARBIDOPA/LEVODOPA IS THE BEST?

Healthcare providers have multiple formulations of carbidopa/levodopa available to prescribe. The immediate release formulation is the most commonly prescribed form and it is the form I typically recommend. There are also controlled release forms of carbidopa/levodopa available in both the generic form and now in a new brand formulation called Rytary. I favor using the immediate release form of carbidopa/levodopa treatment because the responses are more consistent. In contrast, the controlled release form of carbidopa/levodopa tends to be more inconsistent for the patient. There are certain situations when we might choose the controlled release form or when we might use both the immediate release and the controlled release forms together.

The most recent FDA approved formulation of carbidopa/levodopa is Rytary. Rytary is available as a capsule in four different strengths. Rytary also has the same carbidopa and levodopa ingredients at the immediate release form. However, the milligrams of levodopa in Rytary do not equate to the same milligram strength of levodopa in the immediate release form. In fact, when comparing the dosage of Rytary to the immediate release carbidopa/levodopa formulation, we find the ratio is 2:1. Thus, 200 mg of Rytary would be equivalent to a dose of 100 mg of immediate release levodopa therapy. Rytary takes effect within the same time frame as the immediate release carbidopa/levodopa therapy but typically the response will last a little bit longer, which is anywhere from four to eight hours. Since Rytary is still a brand only medication, it is more expensive than the immediate release carbidopa/levodopa and may not be covered on many prescription plans.

Betty Lou's Story

Betty Lou described the benefits of carbidopa/levodopa to me in the office one day. She described the feeling that she had before the medication was taken each morning. She explained how she felt as if she was sitting on an airplane, traveling in coach class in the middle seat between two large men on a flight overseas for twelve hours. She described the feeling of being stuck in this position and not being able to easily stand up and move around. Her muscles were tight and stiff and after a few hours, they were very sore and restless. She described an internal tremor as well as a visible tremor that caused her hand to oscillate back and forth out of her control.

Betty Lou then described how when the levodopa tablet finally started working for her, it was as if she stood up from her seat on the plane and was finally able to move around again. The internal and external tremors melted away. Her restlessness abated and her muscles became relaxed allowing her to walk and move her limbs with ease. What a great moment for her as she felt like her body was given back to her.

CHAPTER 3

FIRST APPEARANCES MAY DECEIVE YOU

Bob's Story

Bob grew up on an Oklahoma ranch learning how to take care of animals and kindling a love for horses. As Bob became an adult he decided to continue in the ranching business but continued to pursue his hobby of training horses. This love of horses eventually led him to the business of horse racing. Over the years, Bob trained many a horse for the racing business. Later in life, his wife convinced him to concentrate more on the ranching life and to give up the racing training with his horses. In fact, they sold most of their horses during the early years when he was diagnosed with PD.

Bob's PD was well controlled with the combination of levodopa tablets taken four times a day along with a second medication that stimulates dopamine receptors called Mirapex. Over the years, the dose was slowly increased to match the increase in PD motor symptoms experienced. Bob tolerated the medications without any perceived side effects.

Then, one summer, Bob's behavior began to change. His wife noticed that he was becoming obsessed with horses. He was researching different racing breeds and going to horse races more than ever. She noticed he was even betting on some of the horse races, which was not characteristic of Bob's personality. In fact, she always knew Bob was tight with money and would have never taken any chances of losing money, especially with gambling. Fortunately, Bob's horse race betting loses were not substantial but this change still bothered his wife.

Later that summer, Bob purchased a new racing horse, which costed him tens of thousands of dollars. He purchased the horses without consulting with his wife and she was shocked that he would make such a large purchase impulsively. Bob was not remorseful when she found out and told her that he was going to train this horse to win races. She told him not to buy any more horses and that she would be watching the family finances.

Bob and his wife finally brought this story to my attention about a year later. They had no idea that Bob's change in behavior could have something to do with his PD and the medications.

I counseled them on the fact that many of the PD medications, especially a class of medications called Dopamine Agonists, could induce an impulse control problem. The most common form of this impulse disorder is gambling. However, other patients have experienced impulsivity for other interests such as shopping, eating, substance abuse, hypersexuality, and other obsessive- compulsive behaviors. Bob's desire to gamble at the horse races and the impulsiveness to buy an expensive horse to train were manifestations of this medication side effect. After I weaned him off of the dopamine agonist medication and adjusted his levodopa therapy, the desire to gamble and buy horses abated. Both Bob and his wife were relieved.

Bob tried to maintain some humor in his difficult situation. He told me that he spent the year training the horse and entered the horse into three different races. His beloved horse finished in last place at each of the races. When he finally sold the horse at his wife's request, the new proud owner entered the horse in the next race and the horse won first place! Bob was at that race yelling, "That's my horse! I trained that horse!" Bob was able to laugh at that story even though his hard work never paid off for himself financially.

CONCERNS ABOUT PD IMPULSE CONTROL ISSUES

More patients and caregivers are learning about this potential change in behavior called "impulse control disorder" (ICD) related to PD medication. A recent Mayo Clinic study found that the incidence of impulse control disorder in PD patients is as high as 25 percent. Caregivers are naturally concerned about this potential reaction.

An impulse control problem can include gambling or spending obsessions. This may cause the patient to repeatedly travel to casinos, participate in online gambling sites, or compulsively buy products in stores or Internet sites. This behavior may lead to substantial financial losses for the patient and their family. Families have reported losing their retirement savings and even becoming bankrupt. Impulse control problems are treatable as the health care provider may adjust or discontinue certain medications, which may stop the pathologic behavior. Caregivers need to communicate closely with the patient and the health care team. In most cases in my practice, it is the caregiver who brings this problem to our attention.

Another concerning pathologic behavior or impulse control problem relates to medication overuse. Some patients will develop a tendency to use the Sinemet medication in an addictive way. We have observed patients with the pathologic impulse problem of obtaining multiple prescriptions for Sinemet therapy from multiple prescribers. They stash medication in different locations secretively such as the car, hiding places in the home, the office, in bags, and other locations. The patient will then take additional pills of Sinemet either with their prescribed doses or in between doses, which may result in a feeling of a "high." The overuse of dopamine leads to side effects such as excessive involuntary movements called dyskinesia, mental status changes, or even manic like symptoms. This may include difficulty sleeping, pressure speech, hyperactivity, and restlessness. Caregivers need to be aware of this potential complication and be willing to report it to the treating health care provider. The remedy is a combination of medication changes, care partner assistance in controlling the medication dispensing, and good communication with all involved.

I recently encountered this problem in a patient that was managing her drug schedule all by herself. She lived alone and had always been independent. When the patient developed this impulse control problem, the family could not figure out why she was having all of the new problems. The problems were not solved until the family intervened under my direction to gather all the pills and to buy a pill box system with a timer and lock. Now the patient became regulated in their motor symptoms, and the ICD resolved. Although this was uncomfortable at first, both the family and the patient were thankful and relieved that a pill box with a lock and timer resolved the issue. Yet, ongoing vigilance to avoid a relapse is critical.

There are many other pathologic behaviors to be aware of, such as hypersexuality. Here, the patient may become hyperarousable and demand sexual pleasure from their spouse or others. In some cases, the patient may turn to pornography. In some cases, the patient may turn to extramarital affairs or seek multiple partners for sexual pleasure.

Dan's Story

Dan was diagnosed with PD eight years before his pathologic behavior developed. Dan was a devout Christian. His family reported that he had high moral standards. He was the leader of the family and enjoyed time with his three adult sons and their wives as well as his six grandchildren. The family had such a close relationship as they all lived within ten miles of each other.

Dan's wife noticed that he was spending more and more time on his computer. One evening, she decided to peak at his computer to see what was captivating his attention. She almost fainted when she viewed on the screen a pornography website that Dan had recently viewed. She couldn't believe her eyes. She looked at the search history on the computer and saw that Dan had been traveling to many different pornography sites over the last several weeks. She confronted Dan about her finding on the computer. He apologized and was extremely embarrassed about his new interest. He told her it would never happen again. Dan's wife kept wondering what could have caused him to suddenly take an interest in this and violate his own moral standards. She was too embarrassed to tell anyone about it.

Over the next several months, Dan became increasingly more interested in having intimate relations with his wife. At one point, he would even chase her around the home demanding an intimate encounter, which she was clearly not interested in at the time. This new behavior continued to escalate her concern for her husband but she continued to be daunted by this behavioral change. On a few more occasions she found him looking at pornography sites but then he would quickly log off and deny to her any wrongdoing. She decided to remain silent of these episodes since the whole issue was so painful for her.

Dan's hypersexuality impulse control disorder reached a climax when a terribly painful situation developed for the family. Dan and his wife were visiting his son's family. While his wife and son were playing with the children, Dan started a private conversation with his daughter-in-law. The conversation started out very benign but then out of the blue Dan propositioned his daughter-in-law for an intimate encounter. The daughter-in-law screamed and ran to her husband to report this horrific situation. His son threw him out of the house and they refused to let him interact with their family. Dan's wife was devastated. Later that weekend, she decided to call me to report all of these problems and begged for guidance on what to do about this. I brought Dan and his wife into the office in short time and we made changes to his medication. Eventually, the hypersexual behaviors abated. However, the damage done to his relationship with his wife and daughter-in-law never fully recovered.

Mark's story

Mark is another patient with Parkinson's disease. He is now in his twelfth year of Parkinson's disease. At this stage of the disease Mark was taking more medication and more often to achieve the physical benefits he longed for. He continued to ride the roller coaster of his medication dosing from on times to off times. When his medication was withdrawing, he became addicted to the medication. He craved the doses of medication and impulsively had to get another dose in as quickly as possible. He would go to different doctors requesting prescriptions to stockpile like an addict. This allowed him to take more doses than what was recommended and he could even take extra pills when he wanted to try to further improve his Parkinson's disease symptoms. Mark was becoming addicted to the response of the medication. He needed more of it to feel good and he needed it more often.

Over time Mark developed additional impulse control problems. He found that he had the new obsession to gamble. He would sit at the casino table and continue to play until he lost all of his money. He could not get himself to walk away from the game. He had a deep obsession to continue playing despite knowing that this was not a good decision for him. He knew that he could not afford to lose the money but could not resist the compulsion to withdraw more money from the ATM and to continue to gamble. Even after losing five thousand dollars in one night within a few hours, he felt a compulsion to keep gambling. He knew he should stop playing and walk away but he could not change his behavior. He eventually lost all of his life savings over the course of a few months. He kept his gambling a secret from his family. He did not seek help until one day his wife discovered this problem. She received a phone call from a car dealership saying that her husband was demanding to buy a car but he did not have the money or credit to purchase the car.

These stories illustrate the importance of care partners maintaining a vigilance for behavior changes through the course of PD. If you notice a change in behavior or interest, please do not hesitate to report this to the health care providers. These changes are often reversible with the right treatment approach. Since these impulse control behaviors were first reported by the Mayo Clinic in the early 2000s, healthcare providers are warning their patients to be aware of this risk and to report any impulse control problems immediately.

Similarly, all PD clinical trials now incorporate a standardized questionnaire to assess for any impulse control disorder.

ATYPICAL PD PROGRESSION

Tom and Richard were both patients of mine. They were diagnosed with PD by their respective primary care physicians. They both lived in the same town and were referred to me for care of their PD about a year apart from each other. Both brothers were experiencing the typical motor symptoms of PD including slow movement, rigidity, and shuffling gait. Tom had the classic rest tremor involving his right hand, but Richard never experienced a tremor. Tom's PD symptoms immediately disappeared once he started levodopa therapy. However, Richard did not seem to improve at all with the same medication, even at the highest dosing level.

Over the course of five years, Richard's PD illness progressed rapidly. He fell frequently due to a rapid deterioration in his balance. His muscles atrophied and the weakness led to dependence on a walker, and then by Year Five he was wheelchair dependent. The muscle weakness caused him to develop difficulty with swallowing. Eventually, he passed away in a nursing home at the end of his sixth year of the illness.

Tom continues to have hardly any obvious PD signs after fifteen years of his illness. The dopamine medication continued to control all of the symptoms perfectly without side effect. Why would biological brothers with PD have such different symptoms and have such different rates of progression? Richard's brain was sent to a pathology lab and the pathology confirmed our suspicion that he was actually inflicted with Progressive supranuclear palsy instead of Parkinson's disease. We believe Tom actually has the classic PD illness with the slow progression and excellent response to dopamine therapy. Both illnesses may occur in the same family although this is very rare. In fact, Progressive supranuclear palsy is a rare disorder compared to PD.

I often hear from families about witnessing a patient in a support group or at an educational meeting that seems to be so different than the rest of the group in terms of how badly the PD illness is affecting that individual. Usually, these individuals actually have different neurodegenerative disorder. We know of many different illnesses that may mimic PD early on in the course but then later, they take a nasty turn for the worse. Some of the names of these disorders include, but are not limited to, Progressive supranuclear palsy, Multiple system atrophy, Lewy body disease, Frontal lobar degeneration with parkinsonism, and Corticobasal degeneration.

If a patient is progressing in an atypical course or if increasing doses of dopamine fail to improve symptoms of PD, it is advisable to seek additional testing and evaluations by specialists familiar with these atypical illnesses. The testing may lead to a different diagnosis and treatment plan as well as a better understanding of prognosis and potential complications to be aware of as a care partner. As a care partner, if you are not comfortable with the diagnosis or have concerns about the course of the illness, please advocate for your loved one and seek a second opinion to better understand your loved one's illness.

IS THIS SYMPTOM RELATED TO PD?

Another concern expressed by PD care partners is not knowing what symptoms are genuinely from PD or from an alternative cause. Care partners are concerned that if they attribute everything to PD, then the caregiver may fail to bring key symptoms to the health care provider's awareness; thus, important problems may go undetected and/or untreated.

A patient years ago presented to my office for evaluation of possible dementia. This gentleman had a history of PD for about eight years and no cognitive problems had been reported to date. His family stated that he rapidly developed cognitive impairment. They described his short-term memory loss and confusion. His family asked if PD causes dementia or if he was in the beginning stages of Alzheimer's disease.

I reviewed the history in more depth. As we discussed the details of the onset of his symptoms we discovered that the symptoms began within a week of starting a new medicine for his bladder called Detrol. This particular bladder medication has been known to cause cognitive impairment similar to what is seen in a dementing illness. After stopping the medication, the cognitive problems cleared completely. This case illustrated to the care partners that we should not always assume all problems are due to PD because alternative explanations may be source of the problem and a treatment may be available.

PD symptoms can be hard to discern from symptoms produced by other causes. PD is capable of affecting the skin in some patients. For example, Seborrhea may be a skin manifestation of PD for many patients in which the patient encounters dry or oily patches of skin typically on the scalp but sometimes on the face. This problem is usually discussed with the patient's Dermatologist.

Meanwhile, medications may cause side effects that may not be recognized as related to the PD medication. For example, a rash that typically develops on the lower legs called livedo reticularis is a common side effect of the medication Amantadine. Amantadine and drugs in the family called Dopamine Agonists may also cause lower extremity swelling. If PD patients and care partners are not aware of this potential side effect, patients may end up receiving a work-up for heart conditions or vascular problems of the leg before it is determined that the medication is the cause.

Care partners and patients need to bring to the attention of the health care provider all symptoms they are concerned about to receive accurate information about what may be causing the symptom. Do not make any assumptions. It is better to ask and receive clarification than to make assumptions.

CHAPTER 4

CARE PARTNER IN INTERMEDIATE STAGE PARKINSON'S DISEASE

The intermediate stage of PD results in more challenges for the patient as well as the care partner. It is at this stage where the care partner begins to transition from a partner to more hands on assistance. Patients experience increasing difficulty with the motor control of their bodies. At this stage, many patients will experience a worsening of balance, which may lead to falls. The difficulty with balance may not respond to dopamine treatment.

The majority of patients will experience a "roller coaster effect" with their dopamine medication, a problem termed "motor fluctuation." A dose of PD medication will provide improvement for a variable number of hours and then wear off prematurely before the next dose has a chance to take effect. During the downtimes, which are called "off-time," a patient will suffer from pronounced symptoms of PD. These symptoms may be both physical and mental. The "off-times" may be disabling for these individuals. During off-times, an individual may not be able to stand and walk without complete assistance from another individual. Some of the patients will experience an "off-time" at unpredictable times of the day.

Involuntary movements, termed "dyskinesia," may also be contributing to the patient's difficulty in carrying out day to day activities and maintaining social interactions. The involuntary movements typically happen during "on-times" and involve swaying or dance-like movements of the body. The movements disrupt motor control and balance. If these movements are more severe, it may be nearly impossible for the patient to eat or drink, perform an activity, or engage in social interaction.

When motor control problems develop in the intermediate stage of PD, providers will spend time with patients in determining the best treatment response possible with their medication. The first issue with medication is determining how much of the dopamine medication they need to provide for the most optimal response but to also avoid causing dyskinesia or other side effects. Some of the patients may be on several different PD medications by this point. As a care partner, I don't want you to be surprised if the health care provider eliminates some of the medications and focuses treatment strategies on the use of the best PD medication, namely, carbidopa/levodopa.

Carbidopa/levodopa provides, without a doubt, the best response for patients in treating their PD symptoms. Providers want their patients to have the least amount of medication that will control the symptoms optimally. The immediate release tablet of carbidopa/levodopa has been found to provide the most consistent response from dose to dose. The range is from half tablet to three tablets per dose. Each individual patient will require a different number of pills per dose. Thus, you should not compare the dose of medication that your loved one is using to other patients such as during a support group meeting. The dose has no reflection on the severity of the illness nor is the goal to move the dose up to the highest strength by some arbitrary time point.

Similarly, studies have demonstrated that there is no advantage in the short-term or long-term in limiting the dose for a patient or trying to save higher strengths for later in the disease progression.

I recently evaluated a patient who switched to my clinic due to retirement of his previous Neurologist. He first developed PD thirty-two years ago. He was excited to share with me that he was taking one and a half tablets of carbidopa/levodopa immediate release formulation four times a day. He said, "I have been on this dose of one and a half tablets since I was diagnosed. Every doctor over the years keeps trying to increase my dose but I experienced troublesome dyskinesia when the dose was raised even as high as two tablets. I am happy at this dose and I don't want you to change my medication." This example illustrates how many patients will remain on the dose that was found early on for most of their treatment years. For most patients, the only factor that often changes is how many times a day (and sometimes night) they have to dose the carbidopa/levodopa.

The second issue with dosing carbidopa/levodopa therapy is the frequency of dosing. This is where the care partner has an opportunity to get involved in assisting their loved one with treating the illness. You may take a week or two periodically and keep a journal at home of several items to help optimize the treatment schedule.

The first item to record each day is the exact time that your loved one takes the carbidopa/levodopa dose. As you are charting this day in and day out you might pay attention to whether the dosing time is consistent from day to day. If the times vary each day, make a note of why. Did the patient forget to take the dose on time? Did other factors such as meal time delay a dose? Did the wake-up time in the morning change and thus change the timing of the morning dose followed by all the subsequent doses?

Second, record the hours of "on-time." This is the time when the patient is receiving a good response from the medication and feels that the majority of the motor symptoms are under at least decent control. As you are tracking the "on-time" you will also record the "off-time" when the medication seems to wear off and now the PD symptoms have returned to disrupt your loved ones function. For example, the return of a tremor in the hand may be the sign that your loved one is now entering "off-time."

Third, it is useful to also record meal times (and snacks if protein is present in the snack) to see how protein intake may be affecting the response to the dopamine medication. The next day, you can look back and record how many hours your loved one slept the night before, which is another useful parameter to chart.

There are certainly some patients capable of performing a diary exercise like this on their own. However, by helping them with this exercise you are taking an active role in assisting your loved one and you will also better understand how the medication is working and what struggles your loved one is having. This will also help you be more supportive with issues like waiting to eat at certain times of the day or not tempting your loved one with a high protein snack at a time when it may affect the dosing cycle. You may also find strategies to help remind your loved one of dosing times such as by helping them set a timer on their phone or reminding them of pill taking time.

If you and your loved one are having difficulty understanding how to adjust the medication and the timing of the medication, your charting will greatly assist your health care provider. Many of my patient's caregivers have dropped off a week's worth of diary charting to my office so that I may review the records and provide advice to the patient on how to proceed.

Many offices now have electronic record systems that may allow you to upload this information to their office for review. Please ask your provider if they would like this information before dropping it off to their office unexpectedly.

One of the new technologies that have entered the US marketplace is wearable technology. This typically involves a watch that is a sensor worn on the most symptomatic side of the body of the patient. The sensor records activity of the patient such as when tremors or dyskinesia movements are present. It records sleep time. It also records parameters that assess slowness of movement and balance. The data is then uploaded into the computer at the provider's office and now the provider has some data to review to better optimize the medication. Not all practices utilize this technology but more options and better technology updates will be forthcoming in the years ahead and may prove useful for some patients. This is technology worth discussing with your health care provider.

ORTHOSTATIC HYPOTENSION

During the intermediate stage of PD, some patients will develop the problem called orthostatic hypotension. With this problem, when the patient moves into the standing position, the blood pressure drops. If the standing blood pressure remains above 90/60, then the patient may not perceive any symptoms related to the blood pressure drop. However, if the drop results in a standing blood pressure less than 90/60, then the patient will experience a light-headed, dizzy feeling or sometimes a feeling of generalized weakness. The patient will likely reach for a place to sit back down when they feel this way. If a patient started walking too quickly after standing up, then the low blood pressure may cause the patient to fall. If the blood pressure drops too low, the patient may just simply pass out.

In the clinic, I find that many patients who develop this problem are completely unaware that the dizziness and weakness that they are experiencing are due to this blood pressure problem. In fact, they will commonly just assume the symptoms are due to PD itself. Further compounding the recognition of this problem is that most patients go to the doctor's office and have their blood pressure recorded while they are in the sitting position. The blood pressure will typically be normal or low normal in this position. Thus, the orthostatic hypotension problem is not identified.

In the PD clinic, the patients have their blood pressure checked both in the sitting and standing positions. This allows us to recognize the problem of orthostatic hypotension. The low blood pressure is often most pronounced in the morning hours. In fact, the blood pressure may return to the normal readings later in the afternoon or evening. Thus, if a patient reports symptoms of dizziness and weakness in the mornings only and they are presenting to the clinic in the afternoon, we ask them to take some home blood pressure recordings in the morning especially in the standing position and report the readings back to our office.

As the care partner, you can greatly assist your loved one by obtaining a good blood pressure machine and helping them record blood pressure readings. I typically ask the care partner to record the patients standing blood pressure in the morning after they take the first dose of carbidopa/levodopa medication. This allows us to understand how low the blood pressure may be and to make proper treatment decisions. You may also record pressures when the patient is having a spell of dizziness or weakness to see if the episode is related to low blood pressure.

When we diagnose orthostatic hypotension, we will then talk to patients and the care partner about treatment options. We first examine the medication list to see if any other medications such as blood pressure pills may be exacerbating this problem. If we can eliminate any conflicting medications, then we certainly try to make this adjustment first. Next, we typically recommend increasing fluid intake, especially in the morning hours to raise the volume of blood in the circulatory system. However, more fluid by itself is not enough, it must be combined with adding salt in the diet. The combination of more fluids and salt may be enough especially in milder cases to bring the standing blood pressure to the goal of being above 90/60.

If the water and salt increase is not providing adequate improvement in the orthostatic hypotension problem, then the next addition may be to use compression stockings. The tight fitting compression stockings that raise up to above the knee level are most effective but may be difficult to put on the leg. The care partner may need to assist with the application of the stockings.

If these conservative measures fail to improve the orthostatic hypotension issue, then the health care provider will likely turn to prescription medication to raise the blood pressure. There are several medication choices available. A medication named fludrocortisone (Florinef) may be used to promote the kidneys to retain salt. In my experience, this medication is only mildly helpful at best and if the medication is continued then periodic monitoring of blood electrolytes are important. A more effective medication is midodrine (ProAmatine), which raises blood pressure by constricting blood vessels. Each dose of midodrine lasts about as long as each dose of carbidopa/levodopa. Thus, a patient may time the two medications together, especially in the first half of the day. Finally, a drug named droxidopa (Northera) was more recently approved by the FDA for the US market in 2014. This medication may produce an improvement in dizziness and lightheaded feelings for some patients, but in my experience, there is rarely a major benefit to increasing the blood pressure numbers. It is believed that the medication works by increasing norepinephrine in the patients circulation, which may elevate blood pressure.

As you help monitor the blood pressure recordings keep in mind that the normal range of the blood pressure is between 90/60 to 140/80. Thus, we would like to see the blood pressure within this range in any position whether the patient is standing, sitting or lying down. If the pressure is going too high at certain times of the day but then low at other times, the health care provider will need to review your recordings and make treatment decisions based upon each individual situation. There are situations where a patient may be taking short acting medications to raise the blood pressure at certain times of the day and then also taking blood pressure lowering medications at other times of the day.

CHAPTER 5

ADVANCED TECHNOLOGY

As your loved one advances in progression with PD, changes in clinical response to dopamine medication may change. Most commonly, a person with PD will experience shorter duration of "on-time" from each dose of dopamine. For example, early in the course a patient commonly starts with three doses per day of dopamine medication. They may easily spread the doses six to eight hours apart without an obvious wearing off effect. However, during intermediate stages, the same individual will find the dose of medication only lasting two to three hours on average. The more advanced a patient is with PD, the more likely the good response lasts shorter and shorter durations.

Another possible outcome in the intermediate stage of PD is that each levodopa response results in excessive involuntary movements called dyskinesia. The movements look like wiggling, dance like movements. These movements may only affect one body part segment or may be more generalized. We have often witnessed these movements as we watch patients twisting and wiggling around. The most notable person demonstrating these movements is

Michael J Fox. The movements may result for some patients every time they take a dose of dopamine medication. Adjustments to the dosing may not alleviate this problem adequately and other medication options may fail to control the movements or may not be tolerable due to side effects of the medication.

In these more advanced situations, patients with PD may be eligible for advanced technologies to help them regulate the ups and downs of the dopamine response cycle and to help treat involuntary movements such as tremor and dyskinesia that are not adequately controlled on medication. These advanced therapies include the use of a medication pump or the Deep Brain Stimulator electronic implant. Your loved one with PD may become interested in these technologies or their health care provider might suggest consideration of one of these therapies. Thus, it is important for the care partner to also understand the technologies including the potential benefits, risks, and alternatives.

It is also important before you and your loved one make the final decision on implementing these technologies that a realistic set of expectations for the possible outcomes of these devices are understood by all. This chapter will provide some thoughts that the caregiver should be aware of from the experience of other family members assisting their loved one with PD using these devices.

When the idea first presents itself to consider advanced technologies for treating PD, I would recommend that the patient consider seeing a Movement Disorder Specialist to receive an evaluation for their candidacy for such devices. Movement Disorder Specialist have additional training to direct the proper work-up to determine if a person with PD is an ideal candidate for one or both of these treatments. Additional testing may be required along with evaluations by certain therapists such as a Physical Therapist, Speech Therapist, and others. Cognitive and psychological assessments are often required before Deep Brain Stimulation therapy.

Once a decision has been made to move forward with one of these advanced technologies for PD, it is very important to fully understand which symptoms may improve and which symptoms will not likely improve. It is natural for both patients and families to assume that one of these therapies may improve all of the problems that a patient is facing with PD. This is simply not the reality.

The first advanced technology that is often considered is a medication pump. An available treatment to administer the dopamine medication more regularly is the external pump system called Duopa. Duopa was brought into the US market in 2004. Duopa is an intestinal gel of carbidopa/levodopa that is pumped through a tube from the external pump into the small intestine where it is absorbed. The tubing for this system enters through the abdominal wall into the stomach through a small hole called a stoma. This hole is made by the intervention specialist performing the procedure. Then tube is then guided endoscopically into the small intestine where it remains free floating in the jejunum of the small intestine to administer the medication. A pigtail twist in the tubing helps to keep the tube in that location preventing it from migrating back toward the stomach. The patient receives this procedure while under conscious sedation or general anesthesia depending upon the preference of the implant center. The procedure is performed as an outpatient procedure. Although the pump is immediately ready for use after the procedure, most centers wait at least seven days after the procedure to initiate the pump delivery in order to allow adequate healing time.

In my practice, patients and care partners find that learning to use the pump, changing out the cassettes each day, and flushing the tubes with water are easy to master. Many of our patients have been able to perform all of the maintenance procedures of the pump and tubing on their own but care partners should also be familiar with all aspects of the pump in order to be ready to help when needed.

Overall, the main benefit of the Duopa pump system is to provide constant dopaminergic administration for the patient to minimize off-time. Our patients have also found benefit in reducing dyskinesia and freezing of gait with this technology, which was not an expected benefit from the procedure. In our experience, the majority of patients were able to wean off of other PD medications, which helps to alleviate some side effects of those medications and reduce pill burden. All patients switching to Duopa therapy no longer have to take oral carbidopa/levodopa pills. Our patients report great enthusiasm with their new-found freedom from the pill dosing. They no longer have to live by the clock as they time each dose of levodopa therapy.

The Duopa pump system does not treat symptoms that were resistant to dopamine therapy. Thus, generally if a symptom such as urinary incontinence or constipation was not improved with dopamine therapy, then Duopa therapy will also fail to improve those problems.

In our experience, the most common complication of this therapy is local infection around the stoma where the tube enters the body. This area is prone to repeated irritation from the tube. Moisture may develop in this area and thus be a great environment for yeast infection and bacterial infection. Good skin hygiene and monitoring of the skin in this location is important. Here as the care partner, you can assist your loved one with periodically checking on the stoma and report to the health care providers any problems that arise as quickly as possible. These infections are often easy to treat as long as they are addressed immediately.

Another issue that may arise relates to the pump itself. The pump is secured on the outside of the body in a carrying case or vest compartment. When the pump is taken out of the carrying case, the patient must be careful not to accidently drop the pump especially when connected to the tubing. This may result in the tubing being pulled out of the proper location within the small intestine.

An example that we have encountered is a patient who places the pump on a table while they are changing clothes. The patient then inadvertently moves in a direction that results in the pump dropping from the surface to the floor. This drop results in a strong force put upon the connection piece where the tubes are connected. The inner tube then pulls out in the direction of the pump and thus the other end of the tubing is retracted out of the small intestine into the stomach. Patients often try to push the tubing back in and reconnect but this causes the tube on the inside to coil up in the stomach. The Duopa medication is now delivered to the stomach instead of the small intestine which often results in reduced efficacy and side effects such as nausea. An outpatient endoscopy procedure is now required for the interventionalist to move the tubing back into its proper location.

The Duopa pump system often provides a more profound benefit for the patient than the side effects experienced. We have witnessed many patients that gained better mobility and a greater consistency of the dopamine response. The improvement in mobility will greatly help the caregiver with less physical burden in aiding the patient and peace of mind to see your loved one happier with the dopamine response. A close relationship with the neurological team is paramount in order to be able to report any negative effects and to have availability of quick appointments to adjust settings as needed. In my practice, patients have standing monthly appointments to monitor their condition closely and at times additional visits are required in between monthly visits to fine tune settings on the pump.

Jerome's Story

Jerome had a history of PD for nearly twelve years. He was still trying to work full-time hours as an engineer. His job required a fair amount of walking due to the fact that he had to monitor many team members that he managed at the office. He had reached a stage of PD in which he was experiencing off-times and these might have occurred unpredictably at times. During these off-times, he would experience freezing of gait in which he had great difficulty initiating his legs to move to walk. He would stand in place, rocking his body back and forth but not be able to take a step forward. If he was not holding on to a walker, he would lose balance and fall. The freezing problem became so disabling that he was forced to request disability as he could no longer work.

We discussed treatment options and after testing he was a candidate for both Duopa pump and Deep Brain Stimulation surgery. He elected to proceed with the Duopa pump placement. The procedure went well without complication. After a week of healing, we started the Duopa pump in the office and monitored him for about six hours adjusting the dose during the time to optimize his response. No adverse effects were experienced and he was able to discontinue his oral levodopa tablets from this day forward.

The next day, he drove to my office and asked me to watch him walk. He walked all around the clinic without a walker and no freezing of gait. He was so happy to have a new freedom of mobility. The elimination of freezing allowed him to return to work. He was able to attend exercise classes and physical therapy. He was able to drive independently again. He felt like he had his life back and enjoyed the independence.

DEEP BRAIN STIMULATION

Deep Brain Stimulation (DBS) has been available on the US market for PD patients for several decades. There are currently three different device companies with a DBS system available. Each company has designed their system with unique innovative technologies but the fundamental delivery of electronic stimulation to the brain is generally the same across companies. Each DBS team at a particular surgical site will select the system and brand best for each patient's needs.

The DBS system is powered by a pacemaker like generator called an Impulse Pulse Generator (IPG), which is surgically placed in a superficial location under the skin in the chest region. A wire runs from the IPG along a pathway from the chest, up the neck, behind the ear and down into the brain. This wire is under the skin and well protected. At the end of the wire are tiny electrodes that allow stimulation to be produced at different locations in the brain as determined by the DBS programmer. If a problem should ever present itself, components of the DBS system or even the entire system may be extracted in an outpatient surgery.

The DBS system allows a programming health care provider trained in the technology to select settings to administer pulses of electrical stimulation to a designated brain region. This stimulation creates a reaction in the brain that is capable of blocking involuntary movements such as tremor and dyskinesia. The stimulation may also relieve stiffness of muscles and treat many of the motor symptoms of PD. DBS does not treat non-motor symptoms of PD such as cognitive impairment, bowel or bladder dysfunction, pain, insomnia, depression, or anxiety.

There are some non-dopamine motor problems such as speech impairment and balance that may not respond to DBS as well.

Similar to the Duopa pump system, DBS is another technology available to qualified PD patients. If your loved one is a candidate for the procedure to implant DBS, then both the patient and caregiver as well as family of the patient should have a very thorough understanding of the potential outcome after surgery. All must be familiar with realistic expectations of benefits from the DBS system as well as possible side effects or negative outcomes.

Immediately after the surgical implant of DBS, caregivers need to be aware that a short hospitalization will be required for monitoring. Typically, if all goes well, the patient will be discharged to go home the next day after surgery. Transient neurological effects may occur during this hospitalization such as confusion or even a generalized convulsive seizure. These transient neurological disturbances are not likely to happen again but may cause panic for the family as an unexpected event after the surgery. The occurrence of such transient effects does not mean that the results of the DBS system will be less than outstanding.

When the PD patient returns home after the procedure, the caregiver should keep an eye on the incisions. Please follow the directions provided by the surgical team on proper care for the incisions including how long to wait before the incision may get wet and when bandages may be removed. If the patient spikes a fever, has chills or other new generalized symptoms, or the incision is pulling open, discharge is noted or redness and swelling is noted in the chest pocket or around any incisions, the caregiver should contact the surgeons office immediately. Infection is a possible complication of the procedure and these may be signs of infection within the pocket or inside the incision.

Typically, the patient is not allowed to drive until they are no longer taking narcotic pain medication postoperatively and the surgical team has cleared the individual. If a PD patient is still working, they will need clearance from the surgical team as to when they may return to work which is usually at least a month after surgery.

Patients and caregivers may be surprised that the DBS system is not immediately turned on after surgery. Most Movement Disorder Specialists and their teams prefer to wait several weeks or longer to allow for time of healing within the brain before they initiate programming. There are more than tens of thousands of settings available for the DBS programmer to use. Thus, the process is not to simply just turn on the DBS and it is ready to work the first time. Instead, many different programming sessions at the Neurology office will be required to optimize the results and minimize side effects. It will also take time to adjust medications in concert with the DBS settings. Lifetime adjustments will be required but often at a less frequent interval.

I often advise my DBS patients and caregivers that the process of programming is similar to starting a new medication. We would not start a new medication at the highest strength. Instead, we start with the lowest dose and slowly titrate up the dose until the optimal clinical effect is achieved without side effects. DBS works the same way, we start programming at a low level of stimulation after finding the best electrode combination. As the settings are increased, typically on a weekly basis at first, the patient will experience greater improvement in symptoms. The caregiver and patient must remain vigilant at home for delayed side effects.

For example, a sixty-eight-year-old patient of mine had just received a DBS adjustment at our clinic on a Wednesday afternoon. She reported excellent improvement of her hand tremor while she received the adjustment in the office. She did not experience any side effects during the session. She went home and felt great for the next three days. On the fourth day after programming, she noticed a change in her breathing. She felt a tightness in her chest that caused her mild difficulty getting a full breath; thus, she felt a little short of breath. This problem progressed to a moderate severity by the afternoon. She had no history of lung disease or heart problems. She became alarmed and presented to her local emergency room (ER). The ER team ran several tests including a chest x-ray, blood work, and vital signs, which were all unremarkable. They could not find an explanation for her symptoms and thought maybe she was just anxious. The patient knew that there must be another explanation for this problem so she called my office from her cell phone while she was at the ER. After she explained the symptoms to me, I asked her to shut off her DBS system with her remote control. Within about five minutes, the breathing problems completely resolved. I informed her that this was a delayed side effect of DBS and she returned to my office for re-programming of the settings. Once we changed the settings, this problem never developed again.

There are additional side effects to be watchful for as the DBS system is being used by your loved one. The most important side effect that could lead to a safety issue is a change in mental status. There are some patients who might develop a depression in the subsequent months after the device is turned on. This depression may become severe and lead the patient to develop suicidal thoughts. In many cases, the patient may not be aware of the emotional changes and may not report the suicidal thoughts to others. Thus, it is important that caregivers monitor the emotional well-being of the patient after surgery along with the DBS medical team.

Over the recent years, the technology has improved with the DBS system. The patient will receive a remote control unit. This remote will allow a patient and/or caregiver to connect to the DBS system wirelessly and determine if the stimulation is on or off, check the battery life of the system, and access programming options. If the DBS programmer enables the remote to adjust settings, then the patient and/or caregiver will be able to turn the power of the system up or down within a defined range. This allows for on demand adjustments at home but all within a safe range of stimulation. It is important to have the remote control with you when traveling outside of the home, even just when going to the store. There are stores that have high power security gates at the front door that use a magnet and when the patient walks through the security gate, the DBS system may turn off. A similar change may occur when going through the airport security gates. With the remote control, a patient may immediately turn the device back on and it will automatically return to the same settings. It is safe to travel by airline with a DBS system. Make sure that you have your DBS identification card with you to show the airport security workers that your loved one has an implanted electronic system in the body.

DBS AND DUOPA TOGETHER

This may be surprising to many caregivers but there are patients who have greatly benefitted from both technologies used together. Both DBS and Duopa provide unique benefits that may be needed in some cases. Although most people who are candidates for these advanced systems only need one system, the treatment team may recommend both after an adequate trial is completed using the first option.

Tony's Story

Tony had a long history of a tremor in his hands. Despite trials of multiple medications, the tremor could not be controlled. The tremor had become disabling for Tony and he needed a stronger technology to help him. Tony completed the work-up for DBS surgery and was found to be an excellent candidate. DBS was implanted into each side of the brain and within months he was completely tremor free. Tony was so excited to finally have his motor control back again!

Despite the tremor control, Tony was not able to wean off of his carbidopa/levodopa medication. He found that the carbidopa/levodopa was providing him with a faster thought process, a better mood, and he seemed to walk better with each dose of carbidopa/levodopa. He did achieve less off-time once the DBS system was implanted. However, over the next three years his medication dosing seemed to wear off after just one to two hours. The tremor would not return when the medication wore off but he was bothered by the other symptoms that remained responsive to the carbidopa/levodopa. He grew tired of the frequent dosing and lack of sustained control of symptoms. He was a candidate for the Duopa system and after this system was added, he enjoyed the best of both technologies. He had terrific tremor control and more continuous control of his other PD symptoms.

Both the DBS and Duopa technologies are not cures. In addition, neither technology has been proven to slow the progression of PD. However, they are very effective advanced technologies capable of treating certain symptoms of PD. Both technologies are capable of greatly improving the quality of life of both the PD patient and the caregiver. However, careful monitoring and thorough knowledge of the particular technologies will be required of the caregiver to best support their loved one.

CHAPTER 6

ADVANCED STAGE PARKINSON'S DISEASE CAREGIVING

ADVANCED PD LEWY BODY DEGENERATION

As the disease advances the pathologic changes of PD may spread into other brain regions. This progression is variable in that not all patients experience more degenerative spread into the higher cortical brain regions. However, if the pathology spreads into other non-dopamine related brain regions, then more advanced symptoms will develop for the patient. The non-dopamine related symptoms most commonly involve cognitive changes. Impairment in short-term memory function, thinking and reasoning skills, and executive function may result. This may ultimately progress to a dementia state where the patient now depends on their loved one for help with day to day functions. Balance and mobility may be more effected by spread of this pathology. Patients may have difficulty with the automatic controls of the nervous system, which lead to blood pressure dysregulation and loss of normal bladder control. Psychological changes may also develop including most commonly visual hallucinations.

Jan's Story

She had no family nearby, so she called the fire department to help her get Steve from the floor at least three times every week—sometimes as often as three times a day. Fifteen years ago, doctors diagnosed Steve with Parkinson's disease. Since then, Jan was the only caregiver for her husband; her adult son lived several states away, busy with his own life and family. She had reached the point where she was seriously considering moving Steve into a nursing home. However, their son was adamant that he did not want her to move his dad into a nursing home. She knew it was time for help, though, because she could no longer lift her husband when he fell. Steve was so weak that he could not stand on his own after a fall.

Jan second-guessed herself each hour of the day. What if Steve would never forgive her? What if this decision caused a permanent divide in her relationship with their son? What if Steve didn't receive the level of care he needed in the nursing home, and somehow, would the move hasten his death? After months of agonizing over the decision, Jan decided to move Steve into a nearby facility. She felt tremendous guilt about this decision. She felt like an utter failure as a caregiver.

Ruth's Story

Ruth and Bill shared forty-five years of marriage. From the beginning of their marriage, Bill was overly protective of Ruth and jealous if she spent time away from him. He was paranoid that Ruth was having extramarital affairs, even though he knew that she would never entertain such an idea. Ruth felt like she spent most of her years convincing Bill that she only loved him and no one else.

As Bill reached the advanced stage of Parkinson's disease, he experienced dementia, along with delusional thoughts and severe paranoia. Ruth researched local nursing homes for Bill after reaching a point where she could no longer tolerate his paranoia about infidelity and constant monitoring of her whereabouts. But she struggled with this decision. Although her adult children supported her choice, Ruth couldn't imagine moving Bill out of their home and living in separate locations. She knew he would never forgive her.

Bill's mental status continued to deteriorate, forcing Ruth to move Bill into a memory center. He had developed an impulse control problem in which he was obsessed with sexual behaviors. He continually demanded intimate encounters with Ruth, which caused arguments and stress for both of them. After the agitation and fighting became overwhelming, Ruth called for help to move Bill into the living center. Medication adjustments helped reduce the impulse control symptoms and moderated his psychosis. However, every day that Ruth visited him in the center Bill shared his frustration of not being able to live at home with her and pleaded for her to take him home. When she denied his request, Bill became angry and paranoid accusing her of having an affair at home and interrogating her about her daily routine. After reassuring him over and over again, Ruth finally had to give Bill an ultimatum each day to either stop asking these questions and accusing her of infidelity, or she would leave and go home. She often left the facility in tears and wondered if she made the right decision.

Steve's Story

Steve was caring for his wife, Teresa, for over eighteen years battling Parkinson's disease. Steve made a decision early on that he would never move Teresa out of their home. He was determined to take care of her to the very end. Steve struggled to care for her when she became demented and required twenty-four hour caregiving. She was continually trying to get out of bed at night. Without help, she would fall to the ground. He hardly slept for more than an hour at a time. During the day, she needed him to feed her, bathe her, dress her, and administer her medications.

Steve and Teresa's four adult children were busy with their own families and work lives in the same small town as their parents. Steve and Teresa's children feared that he was going to have a heart attack or some other health problem from all the stress of caring for Teresa. They knew Steve was sleep deprived and mentally exhausted.

Promises have power. Steve had made a promise to Teresa that he was not going to break. Each day was a struggle; he admitted that on many a day he almost broke down and moved Teresa into a facility just as his children kept begging him to do. The advice of his children resonated with him—but Steve knew that he could not break his promise to Teresa.

Near the end of Teresa's life, he agreed to hire an aid to come into the house for a few hours each day so that he could leave the house for a short break. During this break, Steve would exercise, run a few quick errands, and pick up items at the grocery store.

A few times a month his daughter would come over for a half a day and let Steve go fishing so that he had some time away. Steve refused to give up any other caregiving duties for his wife. He took care of her until the day she passed away at home. He attributed his strength in caring for her as a gift from God.

MY STORY

Every step of the way, the relentless progression of PD drives caregivers to constantly second-guess their actions and future plans. I see it every day in the clinic, and I have second-guessed many decisions I have made in my mother's care. We witness other caregivers making different choices, and so we question whether we are making the right decision with our loved one. The litany goes like this: Should we be doing something different? Will we make a decision that hurts our loved one? Are we supportive enough? Are we paying attention to all of the symptoms and understanding what is to be expected versus a symptom we need to bring up to the health care provider? If you are a PD caregiver with endless worries and feelings of guilt, then you are not alone.

I started this book by describing how most caregivers who have chosen to take the journey do not think they are doing as good of a job of caregiving as they really are. I hear from caregivers all day long in the clinic who share this feeling about their performance, yet by the most important measures they are fantastic caregivers. They put the needs of their loved one with PD first. They give unselfishly, and they pour their love into their loved ones. The best measure of how well the caregiver is doing was from the report of the patient who they care for that gave the caregiver the highest marks on caregiving.

You are a better caregiver than you think—because no one on this planet is capable of caring for your loved one with PD like you. Your love for the patient is second to no other person. Your love provides the security and trust that your loved one needs so importantly.

There are plenty of caregivers in nursing home facilities and for hire to perform home health care but no one can provide the love and care that only you can provide.

CAREGIVER'S DILEMMA

I think the reason PD caregivers struggle in their confidence as a caregiver and question how good of a job they are doing is the fear of the unknown. Neither our loved one nor us sign up for this job. Becoming a PD caregiver was not in the long-term plan. In most cases, we have never been a caregiver for an adult family member, especially with a neurological disease that we hardly know anything about. Sure, we have heard of or seen a few people living with PD, but the majority of caregivers have no real concept of PD and what it does first to a patient and second to a family. On top of that, people with PD continuously get worse, new symptoms present as soon as we gain some familiarity with the current symptoms, and new medications and treatments regularly emerge, further confusing our position.

In the early years of PD, the caregiver is simply a care partner supporting their loved one, who remains mostly independent. During these years, we don't know how much care to provide, trying to toe the delicate and invisible line between insulting the person's autonomy and dignity to care for themselves and offering enough of a helping hand. Do we assist our loved one every time they need something, or does this rob them of the opportunity to stay active and capable of caring for themselves for a longer time? We doubt our caregiving job because we don't know or understand exactly what role we are supposed to do for the loved one, and to compound matters, our loved one doesn't know how much we should help either.

When my mom began dealing with cognitive changes in the form of visuospatial impairments, I struggled with how much independence she should still have and how much do I continue to let her have. At first, it was easy to shrug off the minor damage done to her car when she would gently bump into a pole in a parking garage or back the car over the mailbox as she misjudged backing down the driveway. Later, she would mention near occasions when she barely missed hitting a vehicle going the other way or misjudging a turn and almost running the car off the road. On most days, she drove her little car just fine and only drove within a two mile distance from home to her usual destinations.

I struggled. When should I press for her to stop driving? When do I take the keys away for good? She knew enough to not drive on the highways or longer distances alone. She always avoided driving at night as well. This fear of not knowing how to intervene in many cases was compounded by learning that not a single test or determination from a health care provider or another source existed to guide us on this decision. There are recommendations available from national organizations suggesting we take her for a formal driving test but what if she has a great day and passes the test with ease. This does not make her safe for the rest of the days of the week.

As the disease advances, more care is needed for physical and mental support. At some point, PD patients require twenty-four hour care for all of their daily activities and personal care.

The timing of PD's progression into more advanced stages varies from patient to patient. Here caregivers continue to battle the unknown in not having a clear guidance on whether to keep their loved one at home or put them in a facility with twenty-four hour care. One might have made the decision to always keep their loved one at home; however, circumstances with the patient or themselves may change and make keeping this promise impossible. Some caregivers are surrounded by other caregivers in their support groups who are making the same decision to institutionalize their loved one but the closer they get to that reality, the harder it is to make the decision.

Caregivers feel like they are always trying to hit a moving target. In most cases, the caregiver is exhausted, both mentally and physically. In many cases, respite time is not possible. Health care providers and "Experts" are always telling caregivers, "You need to take time for yourself–to take care of your own health." We are told to make sure we take plenty of breaks. But it's easier said than done.

Many patients need caregiving twenty-four hours per day, seven days a week. There are no breaks built into the schedule. Good reliable help is difficult to find and often cost-prohibitive. Caregivers are mostly as reluctant as their loved ones to be around strangers in their own homes. Caregivers worry that the person subbing in will not know how to handle certain situations or deal with certain behaviors that the caregiver handles uniquely every day. There are situations that caregivers hear about in which the hired caregiver from an agency may come into the home and steal items such as patient medication, especially when narcotics or other drugs are readily available. Even though there are many excellent caregivers available through agencies, these fears plague the caregiver and make some caregivers fearful of taking a chance. And there is the ultimate fear: Leaving your loved one in the hands of someone else, someone unknown who doesn't love them as you do.

THE STRUGGLE TO DECIDE

In addition to the fear of the unknown, there are many other reasons why caregivers struggle with decisions. First, the patient may have different opinions on the type of care necessary, which may directly conflict with the caregiver's approach. Second, caregivers develop self-doubt regarding their decisions and capabilities. Third, family members and friends may have opposing views on caregiving decisions that cause the caregiver to second-guess their choices or cause hesitation in making a decision so that the caregiver avoids disappointing their family and friends. Finally, the abundance of information and opinions available from the medical field experts, support groups, and the Internet creates confusion and doubts for their caregivers, especially when the caregivers receive opposing opinions on the same topic.

Many patients have unpredictable days and even times of the day that make caregiving that much more challenging. The caregivers are heroically helping their loved one battle a relentlessly progressive and debilitating disease. They understand the role in a way no one else can understand. Most health care providers who have never been in the role of a caregiver are unable to understand what it is like to be on the front lines of providing care. Parkinson's disease caregivers see the highs and the lows of the illness experienced by the patient. They see the "on" or good times and the "off" or bad times.

COGNITION AND BEHAVIOR CHANGES

If the motor problems were not enough, changes in cognition and behavior add additional challenges for the patient and the caregiver. Caregivers often observe changes in their loved one's personality. One caregiver said to me, "This is not the same person I knew before the diagnosis during these challenging times."

Cognition continues to worsen causing caregivers to take over more of the daily activities – preparing meals, dispensing medication, assisting with bathing and dressing tasks, handling finances, and household tasks. A patient's judgment may also lead to unnecessary injuries or other mishaps. Patients with PD need more help at night, for instance, to get out of bed and walk to the restroom and back. Sleep time diminishes and mental exhaustion due to sleep deprivation escalates for both the patient and caregiver.

A caregiver who is an adult son of a patient told me that he was just mentally exhausted. He went on to say that after working all day and tending to his family's needs, in the evening all he wanted to do was just get some sleep at night. However, his father, who had advanced PD and was living alone in his home just down the street, would call him in the middle of the night. Not just once but often two or three times. The calls varied each night. For instance, sometimes the call was to report hearing something outside the home, or it was a plea for help to get back to his bed after falling in the restroom. Most of the time, the son felt that his father was just feeling alone and isolated and wanted to know that his son was still there for him. Each time his son ran down the street to help him, he became increasingly sleep-deprived and irritated. His father refused to move into the son's home and refused to let anyone live with him or even consider a nursing facility.

Caregivers are additionally worried about their loved one becoming demented, and ultimately not being able to communicate. Parkinson's disease is undoubtedly capable of causing dementia, where patients lose short-term memory and require help with their activities of living. Caregivers have often heard or experienced people suffering from Alzheimer's disease and worry that PD will cause similar problems.

Fortunately, most PD patients who develop dementia from PD are still able to recognize their family to the very end. Patients may have difficulty recalling a vast amount of information and memories, but they are still capable of recognizing and interacting with their loved ones in most cases. If a patient suddenly becomes confused about their surroundings and cannot recognize individuals, we consider this a psychosis which in some cases may be reversible.

Contacting your health care provider in these circumstances is critical. Patients will usually need additional testing to explore the cause of the psychosis and then health care providers may prescribe treatment.

CAREGIVERS FEEL ABANDONED

Caregivers at this advancing stage of PD report more feelings of frustration. They reported receiving less help not only from their loved ones but also from family members and friends. Many caregivers observed that close friends no longer wanted to get together as often.

Many family members and friends become more fearful of the situation and the lack of knowledge of how to handle the illness so they naturally avoid the situation.

Caregivers feel less appreciated by their loved ones at this stage. The patient with PD is more focused on the myriad of symptoms they are experiencing and thus have difficulty focusing on the needs of the caregiver. The patient may also lose some recognition of what the caregiver is doing for them through the cognitive changes of the illness. Many caregivers expressed frustration with the fact that their loved one did not seem to care how much of a burden they put on their caregiver. They said, "We never receive a thank you for the hard work and caring we give each day and night at the expense of our own health and interests."

Due to the challenges that caregivers face at this stage, caregivers are at increased risk of developing depression and anxiety symptoms. The stress may be overwhelming. Caregivers may have moments of irritation and even anger. The instability and inconsistency of the patient's symptoms and good and bad times create immense stress on the caregiver.

CONCERNS ABOUT PATIENT SAFETY

In our survey, we found that caregivers had several worries about the illness at this stage. Some of the concerns were, "How much more would PD debilitate my loved one?" "Will my loved one be able to walk for much longer with or without a walker?" "Will I need more help to physically lift or transport my loved one throughout the day and night?" "How much will they be able to help me?"

Caregivers have this fear accentuated by the frequent trips to the ER or urgent care to get x-rays made after a fall. Now patients are falling more frequently. A patient will commonly think they can walk safely and leave the walker behind while walking across the room to get something they need. Then unexpectedly, the caregiver hears a loud thud and runs in to find their loved one in agonizing pain lying on the floor. Next, the caregiver gets the patient to medical attention, and a new fracture is found. The patient may need sutures or staples to close up a skin laceration from the fall.

Caregivers will tell me frequently, "I have instructed my loved one not to get up without my help and to not walk without the walker." One patient expressed remorse after a second broken hip resulting from a fall by saying, "I just didn't want to wake you up from sleep, so I went to the bathroom on my own." Unfortunately, that patient could not walk safely without assistance and fell the second time in the bathroom resulting in the hip fracture.

Caregivers are especially concerned about patient safety at this stage. Caregivers are continually changing their home to prevent falls and injuries. It is at this stage that caregivers become the official full-time caregivers for their loved ones. There is no moment free of worry about their loved ones. Many caregivers have been able to arrange for help on a part-time basis to help with carrying tasks, either during the day and/or night. Other caregivers do all of the patient caregiving duties but now hire help with cleaning the house, cooking meals, taking care of the lawns, and home repairs. Some caregivers do it all and are not able to afford outside help.

One of the caregivers told me that she just didn't feel comfortable allowing strangers in the house to help. She especially wouldn't feel comfortable leaving her husband with a stranger to benefit from respite care. Other caregivers expressed concern about how to find home help who did not steal things from them, which included even stealing medications such as narcotics or sedatives from the pill boxes.

Doug's Story

"My wife and I were married for fifty-four years and ten months. About six years after the doctor told us that she had Parkinson's disease, she had been driving the automobile and I noticed a long dent on the side of her car." He asked her about it but she did not know how the dent resulted.

A short time later, Doug received a phone call from their small town police officer whom they knew personally. The officer asked him to take her car keys away from her. He said, "She is going to kill someone or herself because she is driving so poorly." He was shocked by the news and did not realize how much her driving had changed.

In addition to the driving changes, her cognitive changes created a problem with their family finances. Doug's wife had always handled the family checkbook and paid the bills. At the same time that the office called him about her driving changes Doug found several unpaid bills on her desk that were over two months delinquent. Doug had to take over the family finances and bill paying from that time forward.

Doug took care of her all the way to the end at home. Doug told me that he served in the Army for eight years and had played college football for four years. He said, "Being a caregiver was the hardest thing he had ever done." He said, "But I really believe that I loved her more than I loved myself. I cared for her twenty-four hours a day with some help from my adult children."

CAREGIVER BURN-OUT

In the middle stages, caregivers are most prone to other concerns as well. Caregivers report being worried about their own age and health and how the caregiver will be able to care for their loved one in the future. How will the caregiver hold up under all of this stress?

Caregivers may now be in charge of running the family business on their own. They may be taking care of their home or their farm alone. Some caregivers are still involved in raising children or helping grandchildren. How will the caregiver be able to balance it all? Caregivers are constantly concerned about what will happen if they get sick or something happens to them.

Caregivers may get burned out at this stage. They battle anxiety over whether they are providing enough love and comfort. Wives of patients will commonly report that although they want to nurture their husbands and care for them in a loving way, they find that it is hard to be as compassionate as they would like to be. Their husbands sometimes treat them poorly, and the caregivers feel unappreciated for all they do for their husbands. This internal struggle causes more frustration and emotional distress as the caregiver battles how they care for their loved one on the outside while they feel differently on the inside. Resentment for what this disease in their loved one is doing to the caregiver becomes significant. Caregivers become short-tempered, easily irritated, and may lash out to others and even to their health care providers. Our staff has encountered numerous situations where caregivers act out verbally in moments of despondency, sleep deprivation, and utter exhaustion as the caregivers reach out to get medications refilled or disability forms filled out.

Many of these concerns come from a fear of the unknown. Caregivers report frustration and anxiety over not knowing what will happen next in the disease progression. They don't know what side effects the PD medications may cause or what the caregivers should be looking out for. Many caregivers are ignorant about how the PD medications used by the patient perform in different ways, at different times of the day, with or without food, or even which drugs could potentially interact with the other prescriptions. When multiple providers are involved, caregivers can become overwhelmed with fear about how these medications overlap and how to distinguish the drugs' side effects from PD symptoms.

THE PERILS OF NAGGING

Another source of frustration at this stage relates to nagging. Caregivers are aware that they constantly and repetitively ask their loved one with PD to speak louder, walk differently, and perform tasks differently. A caregiver will ask themselves, "How much do I put up with?"

"How many times do I need to say it?" "How many days in a row must I keep asking for the same response?" "Is there an endpoint?" Nagging and repetition naturally lead to caregiver agitation. The more you nag, the less the patient honors the request. The nagging tends to train their loved one to tune the caregiver out. Thus, the need to nag their loved one becomes exhausting.

It is time to ask yourself, "How often did my nagging cause my loved one to change their behavior?" "If the behavior changed permanently, how many nags did it take?" In most cases, nagging does not change behavior. Parkinson's disease results in several automatic dysfunctions that are outside the patient's awareness until after the dysfunction takes place. The only way an event would have been prevented would have been if the patient was thinking about it before the event and thus voluntarily tried to change their actions. Patients are not used to thinking this way. Neither are we as caregivers. When we decide to walk across the room, we don't have to think about it, we just do it automatically. This automatic process fails in PD.

Nagging creates emotional strain for both parties. The patient will be frustrated, and emotions will change. Stress builds and symptoms worsen. There may be times the patient just cannot overcome what is going on. You may think the nagging is effective and will result in changes when, in reality, nothing changes. Nagging also damages your loved one's respect for you. Nagging can become a habit.

Caregivers find less stress if they remember to say "Please" before they issue a request to the patient. You may then make the request as a gentle reminder but not repeat yourself over and over. This repetition is not fruitful. Give the patient a chance to benefit from your verbal wisdom and then back off.

At this stage, many caregivers become more connected to other caregivers through support groups and exercise classes. There is a natural tendency to compare situations. A caregiver may second-guess their approach or the circumstances they create after comparing to others. There is usually little benefit in comparing your approach to someone else's. Your situation is unlikely to be the same and you are dealing with different patients and personalities. You have to find the strategies that work for you and your loved one, not what works for other people.

Your loved one may not always hear you when you make a request. Your loved one may also forget immediately what you said and thus have to ask the question again. Most patients are not trying to annoy you but genuinely want an answer to their question and cannot remember how many times the information has already been presented to them. Make sure you speak directly in front of them, get good eye contact, and try to eliminate distractions. You might ask the primary care provider to schedule a hearing test for the patient to make sure that hearing loss is not a barrier to communication.

One caregiver informed me that his wife was having crying spells frequently throughout the day for no apparent reason. His solution was to sit in front of her holding her hands and then he would tell her the same dirty joke each time it happened. She would immediately stop crying and burst into laughter. He said it was really cute to see how her emotion would change so quickly. He probably told that same dirty joke fifty to sixty times a week.

HANDLING REQUEST BACKLASH

Some caregiver requests are met with anger, resentment, and backlash. It's beneficial to find out the reason for your loved one's response.

Some patients, for example, want to be in quiet and reserved places, such as their homes. If a caregiver wants something else like going out and being with people, then a conflict may ensue. A caregiver may need to respect the patient's wishes. It is acceptable to ask a family member or friend to sit in with the patient so that you do not miss out on social opportunities or engagements. Try not to force your loved one out and create a conflict, know how much they can handle and how much family/friend contact they need. Go out when you can to satisfy your own needs. Share your needs with the patient too. If you feel guilty—ask yourself, "What did I do wrong? What am I guilty of?" If you did no harm and did what you thought best, then you are not guilty of wrongdoing, so don't feel bad.

ISSUES OF INTIMACY

Many of the male caregivers struggle with the change in intimacy between them and their loved ones. Their spouse with PD often has no libido, has pain, and other symptoms that make intimacy impossible. Some of the spouses even lost interest in just having hugs or loving embraces. One of the male caregivers stated that after every time he helped his wife dress, he would ask her, "How about a hug?" This would often break through the barriers and give them a moment to share a loving expression.

The male caregivers also expressed difficulty with patience. They found it difficult to watch their spouse deteriorate intellectually. They tried to allow their spouse to do as much as they could for their dignity but, over time, took more of the control of all tasks from their loved ones.

COMFORT

Many caregivers found that having a pet in the home was also therapeutic for the patient. Some caregivers even brought in a service dog to help the patient with balance and other tasks like alerting the caregiver when their loved one needed help.

Caregivers frequently reported that receiving empathy from their health care provider was critical. They valued a provider that would take time with them, listen to their concerns and needs, and help the caregiver find solutions. They know the health care provider understands the symptoms and challenges the caregiver and patient face. This knowledge helps the caregiver feel less isolated and alone. Many caregivers stated that most of their adult children and their friends just don't understand what the caregiver is going through, and the caregiver rarely has time to be with family and friends at this stage due to all the caring needs of the disease. It is not uncommon for caregivers to feel like a prisoner in their own home.

Some of the caregivers found help in pursuing a hobby such as gardening. This activity allowed them to have some space away from the patient during the day but still be at home and available. Their loved one was given a horn or bell to ring when they needed something, and the caregiver would take a break and focus on something else for a short time. Other caregivers used baby monitors with cameras so they could keep an eye on their loved one when not in the same room yet the loved one and the caregiver still could communicate their needs to each other.

Another help for the patient who has children, grandchildren and other family members living a distance away, is to set up a time to visit via FaceTime on a cell phone, a Skype connection, or even catching up with family pictures and stories on social media. This has been seen to be therapeutic to the patient.

HANDLING PATIENT EPISODES

These episodes are unsettling to both the patient and the caregiver. There may be no obvious trigger. Patients with PD often experience unpredictable episodes of feeling unstable.

These episodes may leave a patient feeling unsteady, out of control, nervous, restless, or a variety of other ways. Patients will describe in these episodes as feeling nervous about what to do. They don't often feel like the caregiver knows what to do. The patient wants to reach out to their doctor for help. They want to know what is going on and what to do about it. There is concern over whether a dose should be added, taken away, or some other provided to help them acutely. The episode will eventually pass, and the patient will return to baseline.

As a caregiver, you might struggle during these episodes with knowing what to do. You will feel helpless and wonder, "What can I do to help?" A call to the doctor's office is often helpful but it might be hard to explain to the doctor what is difficult for the patient to explain to you.

I find that more often than not these episodes are anxiety attacks. Yes, there are circumstances where the episodes are caused by other reasons but the majority of these episodes in my experience seem to be related to anxiety. The patient feels a sense of doom or fear about getting through it. They may also be fearful of the future.

The patient needs reassurance and support during these episodes. Give comfort and love.

Don't try to solve the problem or figure out exactly what's going on at the moment; just be there for your loved one. Give them comfort; find ways to help them relax. Perhaps redirecting their attention to an activity, listening to relaxing music, getting fresh air outside, or just getting a hug and holding their hand might be what they need. When the episode has passed, then you might consider talking to the patient's provider about other strategies to deal with these episodes.

As a caregiver, you might also have the mental clarity to watch for a pattern of when the episodes occur. For example, you might notice they always happen forty-five minutes before it is time to take the PD medicine. Or you might see that the patient watches a TV program or reacts to an article on the Internet and then shortly later has an episode. See if you can identify any triggers to help reduce the episodes. However, keep in mind that triggers may not be present, and these episodes may simply be random and unprovoked.

One patient commonly had these episodes when the caregiver would go to work and the patient was left alone at home. The day would start off fine but before long the patient would develop an episode and call frantically to the caregiver to come home from work.

You are the caregiver from the beginning to the end. Caregiving should not be viewed as a derogatory label for anyone. Caregiving is a high calling that requires strength, determination, and self-giving love. It is a badge of honor. Families should be proud to be able to care for a loved one with a chronic illness as we try to improve the quality of life and ease suffering.

CHAPTER 7

CAREGIVER GUILT

"I hate feeling so guilty all of the time!" remarked one of my PD caregivers during a clinic visit. She said that she is so overwhelmed with feeling guilty at every turn of the journey, no matter what she is doing. The feelings of guilt were causing her so much unnecessary suffering.

PD caregivers commonly experience feelings of guilt throughout the entire course of the disease. Caregivers may experience guilt as soon as the health care provider presents the diagnosis all the way to the end of their own life.

Guilt can give caregivers excessive anxiety and limit their ability to be confident and capable caregivers. Guilt plagues all the caregivers of PD patients that I interact with in my clinic. The guilt may vary in intensity and result from different causes. Caregivers must master these feelings of guilt to feel like an effective caregiver and maintain peace in their relationship.

UNDERSTANDING GUILT

As a PD caregiver, it is essential that we understand guilt and how to handle it. Guilt is a result of an internal feeling that we have betrayed our own values or moral beliefs. This betrayal may result from committing a wrongful act or from a failure to say or do a particular action. When we are not living up to our own expectations related to these values, then we can develop a strong sense of guilt. Guilty feelings may result from our own doing or from an action or communication with our PD patient, family members, or other acquaintances. Guilt is a form of self-punishment. We must find a way to move past the guilt and restore our sense of self-confidence and well-being. Feeling guilty is a choice locking you into the past and preventing you from living life to the fullest.

Guilt can paralyze us or prevent us from achieving our best. Guilt can be powerful enough to impair our reasoning because once you feel bad about yourself, you label yourself as a bad person. Accept who you are, know that mistakes will happen, but don't hate yourself. The guilt will not reverse what has occurred in the past. Guilt can actually help us learn from our mistakes and become better prepared for the future. The patient may show an increased level of respect for the caregiver as a result.

I often explain to caregivers that we need to differentiate between remorse and guilt. Remorse is feeling bad about what happened and thus targets the behavior itself, while guilt targets the self. Remorse can be healthy, while guilt may not be healthy. So, we aim to learn from the experiences and to ultimately forgive ourselves.

Some situations arise in caregiving for PD patients in which the patient experiences an adverse outcome and as a result of this outcome, caregivers may feel guilty for not preventing the problem in the first place.

A COMMON SCENARIO

Here is a common scenario I hear about in the clinic. The caregiver tells the patient that they are going to leave the house briefly and drive up to the corner store to buy a few necessities. They inform the patient that they will only be gone for thirty to forty-five minutes. They instruct the patient to stay on the couch and not walk anywhere or do anything while they are gone. A phone is left next to the patient with the instructions to call the caregiver if anything is needed, and then the caregiver will be able to run right back home to help. The caregiver may feel guilty that they left their loved one at home alone with the risk of injury. The patient is not allowed to freely move around the house because even with the use of the walker, the patient often falls and cannot get back up.

Inevitably, while the caregiver is at the store, the patient decides to get up from the couch and walk somewhere in the house. The patient thinks to himself or herself, "I can do it. I don't need any help, I don't want to bother my caregiver while they are at the store. So, I just will not call this time." Interestingly, caregivers often feel that while they are away that something sinister is happening at the house, and the caregiver's stress climbs as they envision scenarios of what is or could be happening. Now, the patient decides to walk across the room, into the bathroom, and then falls, hitting their head against the toilet and their hip slams down on the tile floor. The patient is in great pain and cannot get back up. There is no way to call as the phone is still sitting on the couch where they left it. The caregiver comes home to find their loved one lying on the bathroom floor, and now a trip to the ER is required to discover a broken hip and to repair the skin lacerations.

Unfortunately, this type of scenario is far too common in caring for PD patients. Patients often do not recognize their limitations and refuse to accept that they may not be able to safely act as they did before the PD diagnosis. This feeling is often reinforced when patients successfully manage these tasks on some days giving them false confidence that no limitation exists. There are some days where the nervous system is not working as well as on other days due to the nature of PD. Now the caregiver is left with an immense feeling of guilt. They knew better than to leave their loved one at home alone, but they really thought the patient would be compliant with their request. They feel guilty that if they had not left for the store, this injury and suffering would never have happened. Those good days fooled the caregiver too.

A caregiver in the above situation may not just feel guilty from their own internal evaluation. The caregiver may also receive a guilt trip from their loved one with PD. For instance, the patient may be angry about falling and breaking their hip and now having to undergo surgery, lying in the hospital bed, and doing the rehab after surgery. They may make statements like, "This would not have happened, if you did not leave me alone!" or "If you only would have hurried home, but you took so long to get back that I had to get up and go to the bathroom on my own." These kinds of comments further elevate the caregiver's feeling of shame and guilt.

This use of a guilt trip can manipulate caregivers and cause them a form of punishment for their actions. The subconscious desire of some patients is to feel better about themselves for deciding to walk to the bathroom and risk falling by shifting the blame to someone else. In some situations, the patient may have felt anxious about being alone and did not want the caregiver to leave in the first place. By using the guilt trip tactic, the patient is ultimately punishing the caregiver for the action and hoping the caregiver will not leave them alone in the future.

We find that patients will recognize that caregivers seek approval for their attention and caregiving throughout the disease process. While the caregiver is always seeking approval, the episodes of disapproval from the patient will likely force the caregiver to try harder next time and put more effort into pleasing the patient, a condition which ultimately benefits the patient.

Patients may even bring up these past events with statements like, "Do you remember when you left me alone and I fell in the bathroom?" This verbal abuse slaps the caregiver with more feelings of guilt. As the caregiver, you are in a position to block those feelings of guilt. It is fine to say, "I made a mistake in the past, and I apologized for that decision. That problem has not happened again, so let's move forward and not bring up the past."

We can control our feelings, including feelings of guilt. You must decide that you are not going to let such a statement bring out any feelings of shame, guilt, anger, or anxiety because you have already moved past the event. You have to make the choice of either allowing yourself to feel guilty or not to feel guilty. It is your choice. Don't choose to continue to feel guilt. Move on with confidence and plan for the future and allow yourself to be at peace.

Another form of guilt experienced by PD caregivers relates to the disease itself. Some caregivers experience guilt that their loved one is suffering from PD and that they are not. The caregiver may feel shame for the way they have treated their loved one in the past or the difficult situations the patient has dealt with in their life, and now they have to suffer from PD.

Caregivers for PD patients will experience a feeling of guilt at least once but typically at multiple time points along the way. Feeling guilty can be a normal part of the process in which the caregiver grieves for their loved one with PD. Also, many of the decisions that a caregiver faces will result in feelings of guilt.

THE IMPACT OF FAULTY ASSUMPTIONS

Wrong or faulty caregiver assumptions underlay many feelings of guilt. The caregiver feels they are to blame for the situation or problems (this is rare). Buying into the fallacy that you will feel less guilty by caregiving "the right way" or by being immediately responsive every time your loved one demands something can lead to problems as well.

During the disease's course, it is easy to acquire guilt related to how we treat our loved one at times. Especially if you find yourself becoming irritated and short with them because you cannot hear their soft voice or because they repeat the same thing over and over. Or sometimes having to repeat yourself because of their failing short-term memory. The long time they take to accomplish tasks and get certain things done due to their slow movements or the long time needed before they can verbally respond to the question may frustrate the caregiver who then later feels guilty about getting upset. The caregiver can feel guilty for not taking as good a care of the patient as they would like or as good as the other caregivers that they interact with. Caregivers may feel guilty for thinking about their own needs or own feelings instead of the patients' needs and feelings. They feel selfish and feel like they are neglecting their loved one with PD.

Adult children may feel guilty for not doing enough for their parent with PD, yet adult children have their own family and obligations. They feel the need to provide their parent the whole-hearted care that they received as a child.

CAREGIVER'S CONUNDRUM

It is natural for PD caregivers to experience guilt by continually asking the question, "Am I doing the right thing to help my loved one?" or they might think, "Am I giving enough time, love, attention, and effort into caring for my loved one?" It is often easy to find situations where you could answer "No" to those questions and therefore feel guilty about your overall caregiving delivery. This guilt often arises when caregivers decide to bring in outside help for caregiving, such as with respite time. While the caregivers are taking the break, they feel like, "I should be there giving care for my loved one." They feel inadequate as a caregiver and guilty for not working hard to spend more time with their loved one.

One of the caregivers told me, "I could never enjoy the respite time away from my loved one because I felt so guilty leaving them with someone else. I felt selfish taking care of myself and pursuing my own needs and desires when I could have been helping them." These feelings of guilt added an enormous amount of stress to the caregiver and did not let them rejuvenate themselves to be a better caregiver when they returned.

In this situation, it is often worth thinking, "If my loved one was a child, I would not hesitate to let them go to a friend's house and enjoy some time away from me with someone else." Think of this situation as: "My loved one is getting to spend some time with a new friend, a situation which is healthy for both of us. This will help us grow fonder for each other. I need this time away to get some things done so that I am ready to be the best caregiver I can be when I return."

DON'T COMPARE YOURSELF TO ANYONE ELSE

Some of our caregivers would meet with fellow caregivers during the patients' boxing class. While the caregivers waited for the class to end, they socialize and compare notes. This is a time when caregivers may hear and observe approaches that other families are pursuing with PD that may bring about a feeling of guilt for the listening caregiver. A caregiver can feel shame that they are not behaving or doing the things that other caregivers are doing to benefit the patient. The caregiver might think, "Those caregivers are fulfilling the expectations of caring much better than I am." This is where the feelings of guilt, inadequacy, and self-doubt enter the caregiver's orbit.

In that short amount of time, it is not realistic to compare yourself to their situations. You do not know the entire situation at their home. Besides, what may work for another family may not work for your family. It is best not to compare what and how you are doing and rather to focus on your own situation. If you happen to pick up some recommendations worth trying, then yes, this is a great opportunity, but don't feel pressured to force changes if the plan does not work for your family.

ASSUMING AUTHORITY

As the disease progresses, caregivers should expect to take on more responsibility and even more authority in the relationship. They should expect to make more decisions, control more tasks, do more for the patient, while setting limits for the comfort, safety, and over-all well-being of the patient, and make decisions, often unilaterally.

PAST AND CURRENT REGRETS

Later on, in the course of PD when dementia is a prominent symptom, it is not uncommon for new and different guilty feelings to arise for the caregiver. As the patient's mind is slipping and conversations are getting more difficult, caregivers often feel guilty for not spending more time with their loved ones in the past when their loved one's mind was still sharp. The caregiver might feel like they should have spent more time in conversations and enjoyed their times together because now they are having difficulty sharing many meaningful conversations or times together.

It is also natural to have negative thoughts about the patient. You might think negatively about them when your loved one speaks so softly and you cannot hear what they are saying. You might think negatively about them when you observe them making bad decisions, spilling things, needing help with simple tasks, and when they make bad choices. Commonly, a caregiver gets even more upset when the patient does something that the caregiver pleaded with them not to do and the patient did it anyway. You will often feel guilty for having these negative feelings expressed in thoughts like, "How dare I think such a thing about my loved one who is suffering from this disease? I should be more loving and understanding. I should think better thoughts about them, but I just can't believe what they do."

One caregiver told me in confidence, "I had recurring thoughts that I wish my husband had Cancer instead of Parkinson's disease so that the disease would take his life quickly and not prolong all this suffering for both of us." She felt tremendous guilt for wishing such thoughts on her husband but she could not help having these feelings at times. But she is not alone. Many caregivers have these thoughts but are reluctant to reveal them. Caregivers may think of walking out the front door and never coming back. They may have outright feelings of disgust. Any of these thoughts or feelings cause tremendous guilt.

There are times when you are sleep deprived and emotionally exhausted. During these times, you may respond with an irritated or even terse response. You can lose your temper during these occasions and then later feel guilty for how you acted. Remember that almost every caregiver has lost their temper on more than one occasion and then later felt bad for their behavior. To respond to the guilt, think of a new plan about how you will handle such circumstances in the future. Ask yourself, "What will I do differently next time?"

Remember that no one is perfect. You can't possibly do everything throughout the whole illness on your own. You may experience the guilt of not spending enough time or doing things together before diagnosis. You can be embarrassed, not like your loved one, and what they are doing at times; you can wish that they die. You may get exhausted and lose your cool. If we lose our temper, it may be hard to forgive ourselves. This is normal. Don't feel shame. You can't help these thoughts. The key is what you do about them.

The guilt only becomes pathologic for the caregiver when the guilt becomes all consuming, causing the caregiver psychological distress, interfering with relationships, or preventing the caregiver from tending to their daily duties. This feeling of guilt, once internalized and chronic, can become a source for both mental and physical problems.

When people are not able to address and tame guilty feelings, the caregiver descends into feelings of chronic anxiety and depression. This situation can lead to an emotional breakdown, and eventually, the caregiver may have suicidal thoughts. If guilty feelings are not tamed or addressed, the caregiver can be relentlessly tormented by these feelings. In my practice, I have observed many PD caregivers who are suffering from the psychological effects of chronic guilt. The three main psychological effects seem to include anxiety, depression, and personality changes. Most caregivers living with chronic guilt experience all three psychological effects to varying degrees.

Susan's Story

Susan would accompany her husband to the appointments. She never smiled and displayed a tense look on her face. I noticed Susan's hands were always clenched into fists, and she would repeatedly tap the floor with her foot. Susan would make limited eye contact during the clinic visits. She was nervous about her husband's condition and asked questions showing concern about what might happen to them in the near future. Susan would become fixated on the worst possible outcome for each issue we discussed. If her husband reported memory problems, she would follow with concerns about dementia and whether she could manage him at home if he became demented.

When I asked Susan how she was doing, she would always fixate on insomnia. She said that neither one of them could sleep. She would keep repeating over and over how difficult it was to fall asleep even though her husband fell right asleep after taking his bedtime medications. Then if Susan eventually fell asleep, she was up and down all night with her husband every time he needed to use the restroom.

Susan was irritable. She would apologetically report that she was losing her cool frequently. She would explain how she got mad at her husband for repeatedly asking the same question due to his failing memory. Susan found that she quickly got angry and yelled at him, saying, "I already told you the answer to that question ten times today!" On many occasions, Susan showed her emotions by starting to cry when her husband reported all the falls he was experiencing and the injuries he sustained. She was distraught. Despite her efforts to control every situation, her husband was still struggling and injuring himself frequently.

Susan had developed an anxiety disorder as well as symptoms of major depression. Her personality had changed, and she had lost confidence in herself as a caregiver. The psychological effects of guilt can also be associated with physical symptoms. A caregiver may develop insomnia. The stress of guilt can raise cortisol levels in the body, which is our stress hormone. Chronically elevated cortisol levels may increase blood pressure, increase the risk of diabetes mellitus, cardiovascular disease, stomach ulcers, and result in decreased appetite.

HOW TO TREAT CAREGIVER GUILT

To overcome guilt, it is essential to work on addressing the guilt in the following ways. First, verbalize out loud what the situation is that you feel guilty about. Say, "I did this act or felt this way because … " Ask yourself, "What did I learn from this situation? What takeaway points may I use to avoid such situations in the future?" Then state out loud to yourself, "What I will do the next time this type of situation arises is … " It might be possible that you will make the same choice but next time you will not feel as guilty because you purposely chose that decision. If you are changing your thoughts or behavior for next time in that situation, then pay attention to what you want to do next time.

Once the situation has passed, and the immediate stress has resolved, it is not uncommon to experience recurrent feelings of guilt. Caregivers report to us that the guilt lessened when they did not blow up the situation in their mind. They accepted the fact that the situation may have been bad but realized that they are not bad people. Mistakes happen. The caregiver must forgive themselves. You might even have to ask your loved one for forgiveness to remedy the feelings of guilt.

It is important to also say out loud, "I forgive myself for behaving this way or thinking about what I did and that I will do better next time. We all make mistakes, but a far greater mistake is to fail to learn from past mistakes." It is therapeutic to actually hear your voice recite these words out loud to yourself. Do it in private so that you will not be self-conscious and notice the healing effect verbalizing these words and actions have on you. Don't make the mistake of saying the words in your head because it will be easy for your internal dialogue to skew the words or add other thoughts into the statements and leave you feeling guilty.

If you did something that may have hurt someone's feelings, such as your loved one, then make sure you give a sincere apology to the individual involved. This is therapeutic for you and necessary to eliminate any feelings of shame. Make sure that you make a decision of how you will behave or think in the future and be sure to stick to your commitment. Taking responsibility and forgiving yourself for the situation that brought about the guilt are essential elements to resolving the guilt and restoring the happiness that you desire.

Forgiveness is the key. You must learn how to forgive yourself and also to realize that you are not perfect. You will make mistakes. You will naturally think about yourself and your own needs while caregiving. This is just human nature. Don't feel guilty about this; it is normal.

You might consider using the word "regret" in place of the feeling of guilt. For instance, in the scenario about leaving your loved one at home, instead of feeling guilty, forgive yourself and ask forgiveness by saying, "I REGRET that I left you alone to go to the store. I am not perfect, and now I have learned from that decision. I regret that you were home alone and therefore, capable of injuring yourself. I will simply do better next time. I am trying to do the best I can in being a caregiver." Remember, there is no formal training and no pass or fail test to be a caregiver. You just simply were put into a situation that you did not ask for, did not receive training for, and have no other choice but to do the best you can with the knowledge and energy that you were given.

A way to use the guilt for a positive response is to try to avoid thinking these harmful thoughts and instead tell yourself, "When I have such thoughts I am going to do a loving act such as give them a hug or a massage or say something nice to them and have a genuine conversation with a loving approach." Don't try to control the thoughts, just move on with a positive response. Remember, you are doing an amazing job with your caregiving, and no one could do any better than you in your circumstance. Your loved one with PD needs you, and no one else is capable of giving them what they need better than you, even if you have negative thoughts or make mistakes from time to time.

In some situations where the guilt is more intense or severe, other strategies may be required to lessen the internal guilty thoughts.

Caregivers shared with us that they had immediate remedies such as going to the bedroom and screaming as loud and long as they could into a pillow so that they would not scare their loved ones. Other caregivers had a punching bag or exercise equipment that allowed them to blow off steam with physical exertion. Caregivers who were capable of leaving their loved one for a short time safely found that taking a walk outside of the home or just having time away defused their immediate stress. A frequent tip from caregivers was to take a few minutes away from the patient and say a prayer for help and guidance. Other caregivers reported a benefit from just meditating and calming themselves in a quiet place. If these difficult situations continue to arise, caregivers should seek help from medical health care specialists. There may be other patterns for difficult times and strategies to prevent these difficult situations from developing.

CAREGIVER SELF-CARE

Caregivers may repeatedly fall into situations leading to guilt that require a break away from the location. If respite assistance is available, then take advantage of this help. You may need to step away and recharge your batteries. Take the time to clear your head and regain your strength to continue caregiving. This strategy will almost always lead to more effective caregiving.

Caregivers reported additional points of interest. One caregiver found relief when she asked herself the question, "What am I grateful for?" As she answered the question in her mind she experienced gratitude for so many blessings in her life. Gratitude has a healing effect on the brain and brings out more profound happiness.

Many caregivers reported that physical touch provided them with a great tool to reduce anxiety and guilt. The physical touch may have involved giving your loved one a massage or simply a warm hug. Even holding a hand and spending some quality time with the patient may reduce the guilt you experience.

FIVE STEP PROGRAM FOR RESOLVING GUILT

When I discuss caregiver guilt with the families in my clinical practice, I present a Five Step Program for resolving the guilt. This is stated as follows:

1. I ask the caregiver to accept what they did or what they failed to do. The caregiver must not try to avoid thinking about the situation because the guilt will fester and grow internally over time. Don't try to disown the situation.

2. Spend some time trying to understand why you did what you did in that situation. Thinking back through your thought process or actions may reveal a solution to avoid this situation in the future.

3. Take the time to apologize to anyone who was harmed in the situation. The apology must be sincere and thoughtful. It is therapeutic to hear the words, "I forgive you."

4. Take all of the necessary steps to minimize or resolve any harm you may have caused.

5. Commit to changing your behavior in the future to avoid such a situation or outcome.

In the example of the caregiver leaving their loved one while the caregiver went to the store if the caregiver follows the steps of saying out loud, "I made a mistake leaving my loved one alone at home. I forgive myself for making that decision and moving forward, I will no longer leave my loved one alone. In the future, I will either take them with me to the store, or I will go to the store when

I have someone at the house watching my loved one in my absence." Then the caregiver will apologize to the patient sincerely. With all of these steps and a plan to follow in the future, the patient no longer harbors the intense guilt and can move on with their life.

CHAPTER 8

CAREGIVING IN END-STAGE PARKINSON'S DISEASE

Susie's Story

Susie was in the clinic exam room when her husband was diagnosed with Parkinson's disease. She remembers the shock of finding out the diagnosis and listening to the doctor tell her and her husband about the disease. Susie held back the tears because she wanted to demonstrate strength to her partner in his time of need. On the inside, she knew this would be the most difficult transition in their relationship and in her life.

Looking back over the years as a caregiver, Susie realized that at that moment in the exam room she did not have any clue about how her life would change. There is no way to prepare for this life-changing role in a marriage. The journey of battling PD was going to be long and relentless. She realized that it was a blessing, not knowing all the challenges they would face. The ignorance of what was to come enabled them to enjoy some good years in the early stages of PD.

The late stages of PD escalate caregiving demands. The increasing weakness of muscles, mobility challenges, and cognitive impairment increases the demands on the caregiver. There is now a twenty-four hour a day, seven days a week, need for a full-time caregiver. Patients are not in a safe neurological state to care for themselves independently and need constant supervision and care.

HARD CHOICES: HOME CARE OR LIVING CENTER CARE

One of the most difficult and important decisions facing caregivers at this stage is whether to keep their loved one at home or to place them in a living center. It's a tough decision. Compounding the difficulty may be disagreement within the family on how the ongoing care should be handled. Additionally, the patient may be adamantly opposed to such a move. Grown children may differ in their opinions on whether the patient should stay at home versus moving into a nursing facility.

For other caregivers, there may not be a choice but to move their loved one into a skilled living center due to the caregiver's inability to physically and/or mentally care for their loved one safely at home. Family and friends may not be available to help, and in-home services may be cost-prohibitive for the caregiver living on a modest income.

The move to a nursing home may be difficult for both parties to accept, especially initially. As I worked with families over the last few decades I have observed this difficult transition first-hand. In almost all cases the patient quickly adapts to the new environment and routine. Caregivers quickly adjust as well. Many of the caregivers tell me the move was critically important and now they are relieved that treatment staff is watching over their loved one, and the patient is in a safe environment with medication monitoring. The caregivers find comfort in knowing that exercise programs and social programs are available at most facilities.

These social programs help the patient to remain more cognitively vibrant. The caregiver now can take care of their own personal needs, get adequate rest at night, and have needed time to accomplish other family related tasks. Some caregivers are able to return to work, others spend much of the day at the living center spending time with the patient but now feel relieved that they are being cared for. And then, they can focus on being with their loved one rather than doing things for them.

Consistent feedback from our survey showed that caregivers wished they had more support from their adult children in making this choice. Even if the adult children agreed with moving their parent to a living center, the caregivers wished the adult child(ren) would tell them the caregiver is doing the right thing. A simple, "Yes, I agree with you," goes a long way in helping the caregiver feel better about this difficult decision. A tremendous level of guilt is associated with this placement process. The caregiver needs to feel affirmed about their decision.

For the women caregivers surveyed, the decision to finally place their husband in a nursing facility was due to personality changes and/or psychosis. Many of the women reported that their spouse became increasingly mean and hateful toward them in day-to-day life. The husband would get upset often, especially if denied intimacy. The wife often had lost romantic feelings for their loved one especially since their relationship had become a parent-child relationship instead of a spouse-spouse relationship. The overwhelming fatigue of caregiving left the wife with no interest or ability to feel the romance. When the caregiver is not feeling appreciated and is dealing with a mean, ungrateful personality in a spouse, this makes the living situation most challenging.

If the husband with PD develops psychosis involving hallucinations, delusional thoughts, and paranoia, the relationship is even more challenging and difficult. The male PD patient may become physically and/or emotionally abusive to their spouse. Many of our woman caregivers report their weak, frail husbands with PD still being able to grab them with a firm grip, or hit the caregiver when emotionally unstable. If the patient is psychotic and has delusional thoughts of the caregiver's infidelity, then a safety concern presents itself for the wife.

In these situations, the first step is to reach out to the health care provider team to rescue the caregiver. In some cases, the patient may need to be admitted to a psychiatric hospital to receive stabilization and titration of medications to treat the psychosis. In less severe cases, outpatient treatment with oral medication may be appropriate to alleviate these symptoms and restore calm in the relationship.

The male caregivers were much less likely in our survey to make the decision to place their spouse in a nursing facility. The men reported feeling protective of their spouse and not wanting under any circumstances to put their wife in the caring hands of someone else. Male caregivers who needed to place their spouses were most often advanced in age, or the patient's medical illnesses prevented the caregiver from safely performing the caregiving obligations.

Many of the male caregivers admitted that their disposition was not that of a nurturing caregiver. Thus, it was challenging for the male caregiver to learn how to be a nurturing caregiver. Many male caregivers did not know how to perform certain chores in the house or how to prepare the meals for the two of them. Many male caregivers leaned on family and friends to help with these tasks and even more male caregivers either hired help to clean the home or to help with meal prep.

Husband caregivers commonly reported that their relationship with their wives had changed from the earlier stages of the illness. Many said, "She is not the same person I married, but I love her, anyway."

Many of the caregivers reported that time with grandchildren and great-grandchildren brought joy into their lives. Caregivers would notice that the patient's personality and behaviors would change in a positive way when the grandchildren were present.

Many of the caregivers of either gender reported that they didn't reach out for help from their adult children because they did not want to burden their children. They would say, "Our children have jobs and families of their own and a life of their own. I don't want to bother them with helping us." This choice leads to more isolation and stress for the PD caregiver.

COGNITIVE IMPAIRMENT

A very difficult problem in the last stages has to do with the progressive dementia. Patients will forget information on a short-term basis. They will often repeat the same question over and over and over again. They may repeat the same sentences or stories. This repetition tries the caregiver's patience. Caregivers quickly become frustrated and speak harshly to the patient saying," I already told you ten times today!" A wave of anger develops as the day wears on, especially when the caregiver is sleep deprived.

Communication can be challenging at this stage. A patient often has lost the perception of how low and soft they are speaking.

Other patients may not be able to speak up loud enough to be heard. Compounding this situation may be the hearing impairment of the caregiver. Caregivers should consider speech and communication devices to amplify the volume of speech. Meeting with a Speech and Language Therapist is a valuable way to explore available resources.

Even if the patient may be heard, the cognitive impairment will often affect the fluency of speech. For instance, patients may lose their train of thought in mid-sentence and not be able to complete their sentences. This causes the caregiver to guess at what the patient was trying to communicate and often leaves the caregiver with an unknown interpretation.

It's tough to watch these cognitive challenges take place. Seeing your spouse lose the ability to work a cell phone, not know how to operate the TV remote, or even struggle with feeding themselves can be very painful for the caregiver. Patients may lose the ability to comprehend the concept of money.

Bathing can be a major challenge at this stage. Caregivers shared that patients often do not feel comfortable with a stranger bathing them. They may even refuse to bathe or forget to bathe. If a caregiver is not able to bathe their spouse, it is helpful to find a nursing aid whom the patient and the caregiver are comfortable with and keep the same person to minimize the patient's stress.

CAREGIVER TO CAREGIVER ADVICE

It is at this stage where caregivers need more support and help from both the medical field and others. Caregivers need someone to talk to, so they don't feel isolated and alone. In our area, a caregiver network was established to allow caregivers to have a contact person or mentor. This person is a fellow PD caregiver who understands what the caregiver is going through. The caregiver can contact their "buddy" when they need a shoulder to lean on or someone just to listen to them. The caregiver knows that this person has been there and understands. Many of our patients have even found small groups that they join through their local church, which allows the caregiver to have outside support to relieve their frustrations.

We asked caregivers at this stage for advice on what they learned through the process and what they would suggest to other caregivers.

Caregivers tell us, "Caregivers need to take time for themselves." Even if this means a short time during the week, respite time is critical to the well-being of caregivers. Many caregivers get upset when they are told to take time away for themselves. They say this is easy to say but near impossible to accomplish. Many caregivers say, "I can't leave anytime because I can't leave my loved one with someone else." Here, the other caregivers would urge a caregiver to find a trusted family member or close friend to help out at certain defined times to allow the caregiver to have a guilt-free time away. This time may not necessarily be a time to relax and take a nap but it may be time to get the grocery shopping done or complete other family-related tasks.

One of my patients said, "I so looked forward to the two hours per week that I got a break. While my daughter stayed with my husband, I ran to the store, finished my shopping, and then sometimes just sat in the car in the parking lot and soaked up some alone time to get relaxed and be by myself." She didn't tell anyone about it at the time but said, "The short time alone gave me the strength to be a better caregiver."

Another caregiver revealed what helped her through these stages of the illness was to get a part-time job. The time she spent away doing something different gave her mind and body a needed break and helped energize her to be a better caregiver. This time away also helped their relationship in that they grew together when at home instead of growing emotionally apart when together all the time. Some of our caregivers had arranged for their patients to be involved in exercise classes or adult daycare services for a half-day while they worked or took time away to do other things.

Caregivers reported to us that they needed more encouragement and recognition than they were getting. They especially pointed out how they wish their health care provider would tell them, "You are doing a great job in a difficult situation," or "You are doing the best you can. This is difficult and challenging." Too often, the health care provider team only focuses on the patient and their needs while ignoring the caregiver. Caregivers usually don't want to complain about their situation or their personal frustrations or concerns during an appointment. They feel like this would offend the patient, cause more stress for the patient, and be burdensome to all. Thus, they remain quiet and suppress all other concerns, anger, depression, sadness, guilt, and anxieties to be strong for their loved one. They also recognize and report that they wish other family members and friends would better understand what the caregiver is going through. The caregivers want family and friends to offer to help and especially to acknowledge the caregiver's daily hard work and emotional stress.

Meanwhile, these caregivers recognize that these same frustrations make them seem selfish. They feel guilty for even having these feelings since they are not the ones living with PD. This guilt is what ultimately hurts a lot of caregivers, especially when the caregivers say, "I'm not the one with the illness, so I can't enjoy the time." They worry and make themselves miserable. Somehow, they need the freedom to take breaks without the guilt.

In most cases, I find that the anxiety and guilt are self-inflicted, and caregivers feel guilt and anxiety without genuine need. In most cases, the patient may be fine with their caregiver taking a break and the patient is happy for the caregiver. In fact, in some cases, the patient needs a break from the caregiver as well! In other cases, cognitive impairment may prevent the patient from even remembering that the caregiver took a needed break. There is absolutely nothing wrong with taking a break at whatever interval you need and for the amount of time you need.

You, as the caregiver, are the source of feeling guilty and anxious about it. This is not necessary. You should not feel guilty; you should find a way to tell your loved one with PD, "I am not going to allow the situation to make me feel bad. I don't deserve to feel that way. It is ok and responsible for me to take time away as long as I find a safe situation of caregiving for my loved one during my absence." You are in complete control of how you feel about it and you have the power to not feel guilty and say, "I am doing what is right and what is best for both of us. If I am not at the top of my mental and physical game, then I am doing a disservice to my loved one as well as myself." Tell yourself, "I am doing the best I can for my family even if no one recognizes it."

CHAPTER 9

BE A CONFIDENT CAREGIVER

HOW CONFIDENT ARE YOU IN YOUR CAREGIVING?

I remember giving a talk to patients years ago and telling the audience, "If you have seen one patient with Parkinson's disease, then you have seen one patient with Parkinson's disease."

My point was that although there are many similar symptoms among everyone with PD, each individual has a different presentation of the illness, a different response to treatment, and a different progression than many other patients. There is no way to predict how the disease and treatments will affect each individual patient and how the course of the illness will develop.

With this reality, caregiving becomes more complicated. Caregivers ask, "How can I know how to best care for my loved one and how do I stay ahead of each turn in the illness?"

"Should I compare my caregiving situation to others, when we are all dealing with different struggles?" Each family has a unique circumstance with a variety of outside help ranging from no support to lots of family and friends to jump in with assistance. Each family has unique financial resources. Some families can afford full-time visiting caregivers and home health aides while other families cannot.

There is no right way to handle each situation. Have you purchased the manual of caregiving for PD patients yet? Of course not, because such a manual does not exist. The majority of caregivers are stumbling their way through, hoping to be doing what is best, feeling overwhelmed with questions and concerns, and feeling guilty about the decisions that they make.

Where does the caregiver turn for help? If they reach out to the health care provider's office or to a support group for PD, the office or the support group wants the discussion to center on the patient and their needs. There is no time for discussing caregiving. More recently, several national groups have organized caregiver conferences but these conferences are limited in availability and the majority of patients cannot attend such a meeting.

Some caregivers struggle because they will have to decide how to handle a situation in a certain way. Afterward, if the result was not what the caregiver hoped for, then the caregiver second-guesses their decision and changes their approach. This inconsistency prevents a good outcome and increases frustration and confusion. An immediate result may not emerge from the first few attempts you make to handle a situation. Be confident in your original decision to pursue this path and stay strong. It may take repeating this approach before the approach catches on and becomes a success.

FEAR OF FAILING

In a common scenario, a caregiver becomes paralyzed by inaction because the caregiver believes that if they approach a situation in the wrong way, the patient will suffer. You cannot predict when patients will go through times of more suffering. This situation does not necessarily have anything to do with you but the disease itself. If you make a bad decision, you will be able to recognize it and make a change. You will have to fail on occasion to succeed. However, failing will not cause irreversible suffering. There may be some temporary pain on behalf of you and the patient but you will overcome this setback and make the necessary correction. The most important step you can take is to make a note of what is going on and why before you can figure out the best direction to take in your situation.

ADVICE ON ADVICE

Caregivers can become overwhelmed with advice. Family members, friends, our church community, or other social groups will feel comfortable giving you their two cents. The more time these people spend hearing about the challenges you face or observe the trials that your loved one with PD is going through, the more advice may pour in. People often have their own caregiving experiences for other conditions and therefore feel comfortable sharing their information with you.

Caregivers tell me that they often receive conflicting advice. They say, "Well, my nurse at the clinic advised us to handle the situation one way, but then several of my friends who cared for a loved one who had a stroke or Alzheimer's disease did exactly the opposite." The caregiver may quickly feel paralyzed by the conflicting advice and not know how to proceed.

Jane's Story

For example, Jane informed me during one of her husband's visits that she had recently taken her husband to the ER when he developed confusion and visual hallucinations. Normally, she could handle these types of neurological changes with her husband but on this occasion her husband became combative and aggressive. He did not seem to recognize her at times and Jane feared that he would hurt her. In the ER, the nurse told her that Jane needed to just say to the patient that what he is seeing doesn't exist and then walk away and leave the room. This way the problem would not escalate.

When she got home from the ER and tried this method, her husband became more agitated because he thought the intruders had taken her away. A friend had told her to just sit with him, hold his hand, and try to calm him down. The friend found that approach to be successful with her husband, who had suffered from Alzheimer's disease years ago. Jane did not know how to handle this type of situation and thus reached out to me in the clinic visit for help.

The multiple channels of advice paralyzed her as a caregiver and sabotaged her confidence. She wanted to find an easy fix to the problem and did not know what to do. We discussed the situation. I explained that there is not one quick and easy solution to this kind of difficult problem. Caregivers know their loved ones best and learn the best approach to try. I asked her how she typically handled arguments and conflicts with her husband in the past. She told me that it always helped if they could take a break from the topic of the heated conflict and then come back to the issue later.

Jane and I discussed trying an approach that she thought her husband would respond best to. She said, "I am going to try staying with him, reassuring him that everything is ok, that PD is playing tricks on his mind like the doctor said it could, and then try to divert his attention to something else." We discussed that a good distraction for him would be to get out a golf magazine or old photo album and look at the pictures together. Her husband loved playing golf in his earlier years. She would try looking at the photos in the magazine and reminiscing on some of his favorite golf courses. She would ask him to tell her what exciting shots and situations he could recall from playing years ago. She then would talk to him about trips they took together by the photos they encountered in the album.

Jane found this to be a successful remedy to his periodic moments of psychosis. This strategy worked very well for them and she regained her self-confidence in caring for him. Jane discovered that while everyone who offered advice may have great ideas and experiences to draw from, her unique situation could not always be fixed by one general solution. She needed to find the best remedy for her family.

Jane and other caregivers often present questions to me in the clinic with the idea of, "Is this the right way to handle this situation?" I share with these caregivers that there is no right or wrong way to care for a loved one with PD. Your caring for your loved one is the important part of the equation. I would tell them to change the question to, "Is this approach working for me?"

Ask yourself if what you are doing is resulting in the solution you desire. If so, then you are doing the right thing for you. If not, then you need to consider other options.

Jane realized that the approach of leaving her husband alone in the room and creating distance between them was not calming him down and resolving the psychotic episode. She realized that another typical time for him to develop psychosis was when she would leave him at home and run-up to the grocery store. During the time that she was away from home, he would inevitably see people that were not really there and become paranoid. He would call her on the phone, agitated and confused. She would have to rush home and calm him down. She finally realized that the only time she could take time away from home would be when she had someone to sit with him and keep him distracted and focused on something else. She asked a neighbor friend to spend a few hours at the house with him once a week so that she could run errands and not worry about his psychological state.

Michael's Story

A caregiver named Michael pulled me aside after a visit to our clinic. He said, "My wife (the patient) is really struggling with her balance. She wants to be independent, so she often does not call out to me for help when she wants to walk around the house. She will get up and forget to use the walker. This leads to a fall. Every time she does this, I get angry and yell at her to not walk without me."

He said, "I came up with the idea that she would ring a bell when she needed to get up, and then I would come immediately to her to help her safely walk with the walker where she needed to go. She did not ring the bell and just got up from the chair and walked into the kitchen and fell. I got so mad that I took the bell and put it in a drawer. She just doesn't listen to my ideas."

Michael was guilty of scrapping his original plan just because it did not work the first time. I encouraged him to keep pursuing his original strategy. I said, "With some patience and repetition, keep encouraging her to use the bell." I told him to make sure she could easily see the bell so she could be reminded to use it should she desire to move from the chair. Over time, Michael found that she got used to this new plan and rang the bell eventually each time she needed something. With the consistency of reminding her to use it, the plan worked for them.

CAREGIVER BAD DAYS

Caregivers have to understand that they will have bad days. Just like their loved one with PD have bad days from the disease, they will also have lousy caregiving days. There will be days when you feel like you can't do anything right. You will feel like you missed opportunities to encourage, prevent a problem, and show more compassion toward your loved one. You should expect to make mistakes and to have bad days. This is simply just a part of the process.

However, excellent caregivers learn from their mistakes. Many of our caregivers tell me that they keep a journal. They write down the successes that they are having. The caregivers make notes of the approaches and techniques that seem to be the most effective for them in working with their loved ones. By writing things down, they have a quick reference point to build their confidence. When the caregivers are expected to make mistakes and then write down the error, the caregivers could review these points over and over again and prevent the same mistake. This approach greatly fueled their caregiving confidence.

Caregivers, at some point, will lose their temper. This event is inevitable. The caregiver will overreact to a situation. This is especially a problem when caregivers are sleep deprived and pushed to their limits by mental exhaustion. Often, the patient's personality changes and cognitive impairment cause much of the frustration for the caregivers. The caregiver loses their patience after so many times repeating statements and watching their loved one do the same thing over and over again that the caregiver instructed the patient not to do. Caregivers may make poor judgments during those situations due to not being able to think the circumstances through well enough in the heat of the moment.

BUILDING CAREGIVER SELF-CONFIDENCE

It is essential to build self-confidence as a caregiver, and to always keep in mind what is essential to the patient. If the patient must keep some ability for independence, then find ways to help them do certain activities independently. If the patient finds it important to have help with everything they do, then find a way to help them with all of their tasks. You must respect what is essential to the patient, even if you would have different wishes if you were in their shoes. You must respect that the patient is going through the illness, for try as we might, we do not know what it is like for them. Help them have the best quality of life by respecting what is important to them.

For example, a patient in the advanced stages of PD found it difficult to be around large groups of people. He especially hated to be around a lot of noise and activity. The noise and visual stimulation caused him to feel anxious and dizzy. He was much more comfortable sitting alone or with one person at a time just calmly talking in conversation. His family was always trying to get him to be a part of the group when all of the children and grandchildren had come to visit him and his wife. They wanted him to get all the attention and be in the center of the room with all the action. In the minds of his family, the noise of the kids playing and running would be therapeutic for him. They continued to push him into these situations. They were not respecting what was essential to him. When he requested to leave and go to his bedroom where it was quiet, they became concerned and thought he was depressed.

I sat down with the family and helped them understand that PD causes patients to have difficulty processing all of the stimulation. It is difficult for them to relax and feel comfortable. I encouraged them to not push him into these social situations, but instead to ask the family to visit in small numbers to let him stay comfortable with as little noise in the room as possible. The family agreed to bring in one child at a time for him to interact with and not to have the large group of kids running around him. By respecting his needs, the patient did much better, and the caregiver grew in confidence that they were handling the situation best for their loved one.

CHAPTER 10

SERVANT ATTITUDE

The happiest caregivers were those who approached caregiving with a servant's heart. They put their energy into serving their loved one with PD as if they served royalty. Every effort was made to attend to the needs of the patient, mentally, physically, and spiritually. In turn, the PD patients reported receiving excellent caregiving.

We found that most caregivers we interviewed approached caregiving with what I call a "servant heart." In many cases, the caregivers were not aware of how well they were performing in this role. To their surprise, their loved one recognized it and appreciated it, even if their loved one did not express their appreciation to the caregiver.

The caregivers that we interviewed reported eight different aspects of their caregiving that demonstrate serving others with a servant heart. The caregivers recognized that they must provide comfort, encouragement, empathy, and gratitude. In addition, they had to be organized, foster relationships, be the peacemakers, and have perseverance.

COMFORT

The general approach to treating any chronic, incurable disease, is to ease suffering and provide comfort for a patient. This approach is especially vital for PD. As the disease progresses, comfort care and maintaining the quality of life becomes the health care providers and caregivers focus.

A caregiver once told me how frustrated she was in that she could not get her husband to go out to places with her, such as shopping or eating at a restaurant. She remarked, "He just wants to stay home all the time and rest." She said, "I don't think he is depressed but he just doesn't want to meet with friends anymore and he doesn't want to do activities with me like in the past."

A servant heart-centered caregiver focuses on both the mental and physical comfort of the patient. When I spoke to the patient of the example above, the patient commented to me that he felt uncomfortable interacting with people because he had trouble with his speech and forgetfulness, which would create an awkward moment during a conversation. He also felt increasing weakness and muscle fatigue, which made it difficult for him when trying to keep up with his wife when she wanted to shop or run around town.

I encouraged her to focus on his comfort. If he is more comfortable staying at home and limiting his social interactions with others, then as a competent adult she should honor his wishes and make him comfortable. Of course, this does not mean she had to give up all activities and social gatherings. She could still be active as long as he was safe and cared for. If he was safe at home to stay alone, then she could make time for her own activities out of the house. If not, then a friend or relative might be available to stay with him in her absence.

Many families have made similar decisions, for instance, when addressing holiday gatherings. If the patient was always the host for the family get-togethers over the years and made the meals, then the other adult children would step in and either host the event or organize the meal prep so the stress would be reduced for the patient. One daughter-in-law of a patient took over the organization of the holiday event. Although the patient wanted the dinner to take place at her house so that she would not need to travel, the daughter-in-law assigned different parts of the meal to various family members. She even created a cleanup assignment. This change allowed the patient the comfort and joy of having the gathering at her house without all the stress of the event on her shoulders.

Another caregiver told me that he felt like he was doing a poor job caring for his wife. He was keeping her at home and providing twenty-four hour care. She had lost the ability to communicate with him due to a stroke. She had a constant rest tremor from PD. She needed help eating, drinking, changing, and walking from place to place. He was spending all day helping her with all the activities of daily living and making sure she was as comfortable as possible. She had no pain or discomfort. He made sure her meds were taken on time.

It was puzzling to believe that he did not think he was doing a good job. He helped me realize that despite being a model caregiver and attending to the comfort of the patient in superhuman ways, it is not unusual for a caregiver to feel like a failure because the patient is not getting better. When we have had to take care of someone who is sick, such as a child or an adult with an acute illness such as the flu, in most circumstances, the patient gets better and recovers completely. This is the inherent expectation that by putting all of our love and care into a loved one's recovery, we should expect recovery and improvement. Instead, PD doesn't get better; the disease just progresses and gets worse, leaving the caregiver with a feeling of failure.

This is where we, as caregivers, have to realize that we are better caregivers than we think. Our expectations have to change. My caregiver friend was providing comfort for her each day and night. He was lessening the burden on her and helping her with all her needs. He was turning her, so she wouldn't be uncomfortable at night in bed. He was a fantastic caregiver in providing comfort to his loved one.

He remarked, "I promised her when we got married that I would always take care of her and never put her in a nursing home, if she was ill."

Caregiving is selfless giving. You have to commit to this oath, for better or worse, and find peace in your decision. You will have times that you wish you never agreed to be the caregiver, but once you sign on, you must move forward. If you are a spouse, you will likely not have a choice. This is part of the wedding vows. If you are an adult child, relative, or friend, then you may have more choice in the matter. Even a spouse may choose to just move you into a nursing facility and let the staff be the twenty-four hour caregiver. In some cases, there is no other alternative because you are unable to care for them safely due to your own health situation or other life situation.

ENCOURAGEMENT

Every year in our local community, a statewide nonprofit organization supporting the PD community hosts a 5K walk/run event. A patient who used to run road races when he was younger could no longer run in races after twelve years of PD. He could still walk independently. His family, consisting of five grown children, their families, and his wife, decided to come together and participate in the event. The family had t-shirts made with their PD loved one's name on the back of the shirt, showing that they were all part of his team.

The family, including all of the grandchildren, showed up with the patient each year for the event. They huddled around him and gave him cheers and applauded him walking along the route. They walked every mile with him cheering him along. You could see the joy in his eyes and the pride he had knowing that his family was encouraging him and loving him all the way. The love and support were palpable.

Every day in the clinic I see adult children, sons and daughters, and even grandchildren coming to their appointments to encourage their loved ones and show support. They hear about the importance of exercise and being consistent with taking medication on time. They leave the appointment ready to encourage their loved one to do what is needed to battle the disease. Even if a family does not live in the same area or town, they can still encourage the caregiver and patient from afar. Using Skype or FaceTime, families can call and just by a short visit give a patient and caregiver the encouragement to keep fighting!

EMPATHY

To be an effective caregiver, we must develop empathy. A person with PD needs sincere emotional support throughout the journey as the disease progresses. It is essential to spend quality time together and engage in conversations as long as the patient can do so.

Try to understand how your loved one is feeling throughout the journey. Just because they told you how they were feeling last year or a few months ago doesn't mean their feelings haven't changed. Don't assume you know how they feel by the way they look or even when they placate you with "I'm doing fine." Internally, they may not be "fine."

Caregivers with PD patients often find that they have a strong motivation to conceal their suffering to avoid burdening others. Sharing our feelings creates vulnerability. There may be times when patients are more willing to share and other times when they need some space. As a caregiver for your loved one, no one will know how to differentiate these times better that you.

The best way to empathize with someone with PD is to engage in a meaningful conversation and listen to how they are feeling. Don't try to talk them out of how they feel.

Don't disagree with them, and importantly, you don't need to try to fix anything. Just listen! Put away the distractions, make eye contact, and show them that you are listening attentively and sincerely. When the person with PD feels that they are being heard, they experience great comfort about their suffering. You do your best service to them by just being willing to listen and empathize with how they are feeling.

PEACEMAKERS

One of the goals of serving your loved one is to be a peacemaker. Aim to build teams with friends, family, and medical professionals. Keep positive relationships and try to shield your loved one from limited or no exposure to negative relationships. You may have to work on strained relationships or fractured relationships. Keep stressful relationships to a minimum. Help them navigate the relationships and events in a positive way.

Joe shared with me a concern regarding his wife's symptom "flare-ups." She would have many good days when her symptoms appeared well controlled on the current medication. However, she seemed to have episodic days when her tremor would be present in all four limbs and quite severe. She would have trouble walking during these times and needed help with her activities of daily living.

As Joe and I explored the situation by thinking through any provoking factors he realized it always correlated with days that their adult daughter would ask them to babysit their grandchildren. Joe's wife with PD would not be able to handle the stress of keeping the grandchildren, and she knew that it was not safe for her and Joe to try to watch them all day long. However, her daughter would not accept "No" from her parents. Ultimately, she didn't want her in-laws to watch her children, so she forced her parents to take the job even though her parents couldn't handle it. Their daughter would not discuss the situation and would not accept their explanation.

Joe decided to ask me to write a letter to the adult daughter informing her that they could no longer be asked to babysit the grandkids. Due to the stress her mother's PD was exacerbated and flared up. I happily wrote the letter and sent it to them. At the next visit, Joe told me how happy they were. The daughter did not realize what a problem this was causing and she decided to find an alternative babysitter. She was not upset with her parents and accepted the course of action. The stress was lifted from Joe's wife and now her PD did not flare up as before. Joe found a way to maintain peace in his family by asking me to intervene on their behalf.

Throughout caregiving, there will be moments when pride and arrogance get in the way.

We must humble ourselves as caregivers and serve our loved ones as we would want to be served. We learn to shift the focus away from ourselves. The prime focus is on the patient, and we are secondary. Even if we do not receive thanks and praise from our dedicated service, we must not let that reality sway us from the job at hand.

RELATIONSHIPS

People with Parkinson greatly benefit from the services provided by their health care team. This includes not only the Health Care Providers but also the Speech Pathologists, Physical Therapists, Occupational Therapists, Social Workers, Dieticians, Counselors, and others. As caregivers, we help our loved one with PD to find the appropriate medical team to help the loved one receive the best possible care.

Our best caregivers would always work hard to maintain these relationships. They made sure the patient showed up on time for appointments and took notes for the patient on any recommendations or follow through suggested so that the caregiver could help the patient succeed. They always thanked the providers and showed gratitude for the expertise the providers shared with them. In situations where the loved one with Parkinson did not get along as well, let us say with a particular therapist, then the caregiver would either help find a different provider that would maintain a more positive relationship or try to help improve the existing relationship.

A daughter of one of our patients became stressed over the demands of caregiving and the frustrations of sleepless nights. If there were any delays in getting her father's medication refilled from the pharmacy, then she would call our office and chew out the staff. The outlet to her frustrations became the medical office's. On several occasions, when she needed disability paperwork completed, if the paperwork was not completed within twenty-four hours, she became hostile and abusive to our office. She walked into our office waiting room and loudly shouted at the front desk receptionist in anger about the paperwork not ready for pick-up. The patients and families in the waiting room were in shock, listening to her tirade. She made threats of hurting people in our office and sputtering threats such as, "I am going to kill him if this isn't done today!" We had to call for security to have her removed and her father was dismissed from the practice because despite multiple warnings and letters about her inappropriate behavior, she refused to change and continued her abusive behavior.

This is an extreme example of how the stress of caregiving can make people react in a terrible way. What is more commonly experienced from caregivers is rude, inappropriate comments or behaviors on the phone while discussing problems with the medical office. This negativity and poor behavior do not help build the positive relationship needed for the patient.

The caregivers that behave this way end up sabotaging the care of their loved ones. Your medical office staff is not the punching bag for caregivers to relieve their stress and frustrations.

Some patients can become dependent on their caregivers and discontinue tasks they are capable of performing independently. Patients can become entirely dependent on their caregivers earlier than necessary. As the patient becomes habituated to the caregiver performing all of their daily tasks the patient becomes less motivated to be independent. Before long, the patient becomes like a child dependent upon their parent for care. Some patients enjoy having someone else care for them, and then they can avoid other household duties. Some patients desire to help but are physically and/or mentally limited. Not being allowed to help takes away the patients' sense of worth and well-being. Patients lose the pleasure of contributing to the family. The patient loses self-worth and self-esteem.

ORGANIZATION

A caregiver can significantly help their loved one with PD by staying organized and prepared for each visit. Over the years that a patient battles PD, a plethora of medications will have been used, and numerous visits to different health care providers will be completed. Besides, there will be endless test results and evaluations performed that will create important data. Organized caregivers will often carry a binder full of records, test results, and key information with copies so that any health care provider will have all the data that the health care provider might need.

If the caregiver can keep a running list of medications tried and failed with dates that match the medication's use and the date that the patient stopped using the medicine, then the providers will have a much easier time helping the caregiver and patient. If the patient experienced allergies or intolerance to certain medications, then charting these findings is vital.

Keep a list of all health care providers and all test results. Jot down notes from the visits so that the patient can remember the visit's details. Be your loved one's secretary because they will not be able to remember all the details discussed at the appointment.

The caregiver should keep track of the dates of appointments, treatments, and procedures. Make sure you keep a calendar of appointments to give the patient the confidence that care is organized, and they will not forget anything. Similarly, keeping track of refills and delivery times of medications may also be beneficial.

PERSEVERANCE

One caregiver told me, "This is not a sprint; this is like running a marathon!" He was referring to caregiving for PD. He knew that he would have to be mentally, physically, and emotionally prepared for the journey. He prepared by making sure that he maintained a healthy diet, regularly exercised, and had respite times built into the weekly schedule where his family would help him get away for a break. He scheduled regular fishing trips to be able to have some alone time and time to regain his strength to be the best caregiver he could be.

Caregiving is perhaps the hardest work on the planet. It is mentally and physically exhausting. You will get little to no thanks or personal recognition for your work. There is no pay or benefits for your hard hours worked. There is no trophy or medal to honor you. Your honor will come after this life when your God rewards you for putting others first, for loving someone more than yourself, and giving in a servant way. Many people get strength and feel the reward from their spiritual beliefs.

GRATITUDE

Be grateful for this opportunity to serve as a PD caregiver to your loved one. Grateful caregivers are better caregivers. They tend to be more compassionate, less resentful about their sacrifices, and more empathetic. Show people and the patient how much you appreciate your loved one and what they are dealing with. Always be authentic, avoid generalities, and tell people specifically what you appreciate. Being grateful reduces the opportunity to become angry or jealous. Thus, you will feel better, and you will be a better caregiver. Gratitude will lead you toward trusting and confident relationships. Gratitude will allow you to accomplish more as the caregiver. The wrong attitude for the caregiver is the idea that the patient should be grateful for their help, "For all the blood, sweat and tears I shed to help them." Instead, be grateful to have an opportunity to aid the patient.

Show appreciation for the patient's positive actions. Think of creative ways to celebrate, such as a celebration with cake and ice cream, or try a special prize after consistently attending an exercise class for a month or six months. Share with the patient what inspires you about their approach to the disease and their accomplishments.

If you find you are thankful for the time that you share with the patient, the time you can never get back, then make memories. You will naturally desire to spend time again together in the future. This leads to better caregiving. Other people will appreciate your gratitude and continue to want to help and support you and the patient.

You did not have a class to learn to be a caregiver. So instead of fighting the situation or being upset about it, keep thinking yourself, "How will being a caregiver to my family member with PD be a good experience for me? What good things will possibly happen from this situation?"

True humility is thinking less about your needs. Now we can better serve others when we forget our needs. Lots of experts and providers tell caregivers to make sure that their focus is on their needs and make sure they are attended too. Some caregivers are serving their own personal achievement or personal recognition needs. This is manipulating the patient, not serving others.

We are all naturally selfish. Our culture teaches and expects us to be selfish and do what feels good. To be a servant caregiver, you must, by definition, have self-denial and put your loved one's needs first. This is very hard to accomplish.

Don't compare, compete, or critique other caregivers. Focus on your own caregiving. All situations are unique. Instead of wasting time on these battles, spend time giving care to your loved one. Don't think of caregiving as a penalty or a job you are forced to do but instead see it as a wonderful opportunity to do something extraordinary. Albert Schweitzer said, "The only really happy people are those who have learned how to serve."

CHAPTER 11

OFFERING HOPE

"Hope sees the invisible, feels the intangible and achieves the impossible."

—Mother Teresa

Hope is the greatest gift a caregiver can give a loved one with PD. It's hope that provides the strength to cope with adversities of the disease and provides the determination to live for the future. Hope can come from within the patient or from outside. Patients need their caregivers to validate their sense of hope. Find out how much hope the patient has. Find out what hope they genuinely feel and where they draw their strength to persevere.

Sally's Story

When Sally received the news about the diagnosis of PD, she immediately turned to books and the Internet to research the condition. To her dismay, she learned that there is no cure or treatment to slow down the progression of the illness. Sally read about helpful treatments that would lose efficacy over time. She read about the progressive disability caused by the disease and the complications she may one day face.

Sally slowly lost hope in the future. She saw her future as dark and hopeless. Sally became depressed and lost interest in many of the activities she enjoyed. Her husband, the caregiver, was trying to find any way possible to cheer her up and to encourage her to persevere.

Eventually, her husband, after talking to other people at a support group meeting, learned that a clinical trial with the potential to slow down the disease progression had opened at a nearby facility. He made a call to the clinic and spoke to the Research Coordinator. He learned Sally might be a candidate for the clinical trial. He set up an appointment for her to screen for the clinical trial and they went to the appointment together. Sally was accepted for the trial and started the treatment. Even though she knew there was no guarantee that the medication would work, Sally now found hope for a better future. The caregiver shared with me what a difference having hope made in Sally's life and how her entire outlook and zest for life changed.

FIVE STRATEGIES FOR BUILDING HOPE

Caregivers play a crucial role in increasing hope for their loved ones. There are five critical strategies for the caregiver to build hope opportunities for their loved one. The first is to make the patient feel important. As the disease advances, it is easy to talk over the patient, especially to friends in social settings or with the patient's doctor. Caregivers are often trying to help their loved one by not making them have to tell the story or provide the update. Meanwhile, this may cause the patient to feel unimportant. A patient may feel isolated as if they have no use in the social gathering or, even worse, no purpose in life anymore.

Many caregivers in my practice do an excellent job of letting the patient try to tell me all that is on their mind. They try not to jump in and answer questions unless the caregiver is asked a question directly. Caregivers will often ask the patient repeatedly throughout the interview if they have any more questions or problems they want to discuss to keep the patient in the center of the visit and to let the patient know how important they are.

As a provider, it would often be much easier and faster to walk into a clinic visit and go directly to the caregiver to receive the immediate update on the condition, hear about what problems need to be addressed, or how a medication is either working or not working from the last visit. The caregiver is capable of responding quickly and thoroughly to allow more information and topics to be discussed. I always try to start with the patient first. I want to learn how they are feeling. The patient should feel important, and their report should be the most important. I want to know what questions they have and their opinion on each step of the treatment plan. This is paramount to providing the patient with hope.

The second strategy is to help patients maintain meaningful relationships. It's important that caregivers provide opportunities for the patient to socialize and spend time with family members and close friends. Often, a patient may have had a previous marriage, and their children are of adult age. The new spouse, who is the current caregiver, may not feel motivated to make sure the stepchildren have opportunities to maintain a strong and close relationship with the patient. Even if in-person visits are not frequently possible, phone calls, Skype, or FaceTime connections provide vital opportunities to maintain these relationships, which further builds hope for the patient.

Humor offers a third strategy. A caregiver should look for opportunities to bring humor into the daily routine. It is critical to always be respectful and not make light of things that will upset the patient. However, laughter is not only a good medicine for both the patient and caregiver, but humor builds hope and great memories for the patient. Find ways to make memories, including times of laughter and fun. Don't be afraid to reminisce about fun times in the past that can bring a chuckle or even a belly laugh to the patient as you remember those fun events.

One of the caregivers in our practice shared with us that she kept a notebook of funny events or humorous statements that were shared between the caregiver and the patient. When the patient would say something funny, that brought light to an otherwise stressful moment dealing with PD symptoms, she would write down the story. Then periodically, when her husband with PD was feeling particularly sad, she would read some of the stories from the notebook, and they would share laugh after laugh!

The fourth strategy is to set realistic goals as a team in living with PD. If you feel that the patient has an expectation that is not realistic, don't be afraid to set new goals that are more realistic to the stage of the PD. Once you agree on those goals, it gives the patient renewed hope in the future with the possibility of achieving those goals and having something to look forward to.

Nurturing hope is the fifth and final strategy. Unfortunately, the caregiver may instead reduce hope for the patient. If the caregiver devalues the patient, isolates the patient, fails to help set goals for the patient, and does not support the patient for receiving treatment for pain and other symptoms, the patient may lose hope.

Helping the patient achieve relief from PD's significant symptoms can bring hope to the patient. When the patient sees that a remedy for a particular symptom is available and the patient responds to the treatment, the patient will naturally build hope that they can fight this illness. If you and the patient are finding that some of the symptoms are not being adequately addressed, don't be afraid to keep pushing for help.

For example, many Neurologists are uncomfortable discussing psychological symptoms of PD, such as depression or anxiety. This is not their real specialty; thus, they may choose to focus on motor symptoms such as tremor, gait impairment, and balance. If the depression or anxiety symptoms are not brought to their attention, the Neurologist may not ask. They may also feel that the primary care physician or provider is addressing these symptoms and therefore the Neurologist only needs to concentrate on the motor symptoms. Meanwhile, the primary care team may be deferring treatment and discussion of these psychological symptoms to the treating Neurologists. If you recognize that depression or other psychiatric symptoms are significantly affecting the patient's quality of life and needs to be treated, please bring this problem up to the providers. If they do not take it seriously, then call their office after the visit and request a referral to a psychiatrist or psychologist to formally address these problems if the patient is comfortable with this approach.

Don't be afraid to keep pushing until someone listens and provides help. A recent study found that depression symptoms can cause the most impairment of quality of life for patients, yet this may be one of the least evaluated symptoms by the health care provider team. Fortunately, my study's result has led to a shift in awareness, and more providers are now discussing depression and other psychological symptoms with their patients. Many providers are even asking the patient to fill out a depression screening test to look for evidence of depression.

The caregiver can focus on what is possible to happen through the course of the disease and help eliminate unreasonable fears. You can emphasize and remind the patient that inner peace is possible at any stage of the disease. Give them hope that they can rise to the challenge or obstacle directly ahead and overcome this challenge. There are times when your loved one needs you to point out the silver lining in a difficult situation. You can help them realize that despite their challenges, they can still have a positive effect on other people. They can try to live the best they can in all circumstances.

SOURCES OF HOPE

Hope comes from what matters most to the patient and caregiver. Find out what matters most to the patient. Find out what the patient truly values. You might be surprised by the answer. For example, their most important value may be living the rest of the way with PD without pain. Perhaps they wish to keep living until they can witness a family member's wedding day or graduation ceremony. Maybe they want to live to meet a new grandchild or great grandchild.

Some patients may find hope in achieving the goal of not being a burden to their family. Some patients have a bucket list and see there are specific goals and achievements left to strive for. Other patients may desire to leave a legacy. Achieving closure to certain aspects of their life to leave such a legacy may be the primary concern of the patient, not entirely relieving a tremor as their doctor may believe. Help your loved one find their goals and help them develop a plan. Your assistance in finding out what their life values are now that the disease has been accepted can provide tremendous hope for the patient.

Another helpful tool in building hope for the patient is to help them to communicate with other patients. They may resist the idea of going to support groups or exercise groups.

However, the patient will often go if the caregiver encourages them to go together and have time to communicate with other patients. This excursion offers a valuable time for the caregivers to communicate with each other and learn secrets and attain support that is so dearly needed.

A great way to inspire hope is to generously listen to the patient. Don't assume you know all about how the patient feels, and there is nothing more you can learn from interacting with them. Instead, always actively listen to your loved one and be available and supportive of them. Give them time to communicate and don't rush to finish their sentences or thoughts, and don't allow yourself to get distracted with other things. Genuinely listen with great interest.

Hope prevents a patient from dipping into a state of utter despair. Even in the end stages, PD patients need hope for the dying process. Even hope in life after death can be crucial to the patient. Hope comes from an affirmative acceptance of the future of the disease. Anticipating the positive future of the disease is not the worst. In the end stages, people tend to avoid patients because they don't know what to say. Just go in and talk about something and listen. This action reassures the patient that someone is there for them. Give your loved one a chance to say it's a bad day and give them a chance to hope for a better tomorrow.

Hope is a response to a threat. Helplessness, isolation and fear strangle hope. Psychological therapy can be a vital tool for both patients and caregivers. Caregivers need to acknowledge their feelings. The old method was to withhold information and the prognosis to protect the emotions of the patient and not to take away hope. However, we find in my practice that this action actually causes more difficulty for patients because they cannot plan for the future. Maintain open communication.

Hope is a dynamic process at all stages of the illness. Changing events along the course of the disease can affect your loved one's hope. Help your loved one to set goals, think positive self thoughts, rethink a realistic future, explore their spirituality and next life, come to find peace, and find ways to increase energy.

Hopelessness leads to decreased physical health, depression, and even thoughts of suicide. It can be challenging to have hope with this disease. You have to feed the patient's hope. Caregivers need to stay engaged with the patient. Set attainable goals (like exercise, spiritual, etc.), comfort them, support their spiritual needs and relationships, and seek humor. Shift their perspective (and yours) from dying from PD to living with PD. Ease the physical burden by using a scooter or electric wheelchair. Maintain good caring relationships, make them feel valued.

Hope helps the caregiver cope. If caregivers have hope, their hope helps the patient have hope. Caregivers need to deal with grief and learn coping strategies to improve their hope and to cope with the eventual loss.

The spirituality of the patient and caregiver is an essential aspect of hope. Hope can lie in the transcendent meaning of life. Strong spiritual beliefs offer a compelling way to deal with PD. Spirituality may also help a caregiver deal with grief.

CHAPTER 12

PEACEFUL CAREGIVING

PLS "PLEASE" METHOD (PATIENCE, LEADERSHIP, SERVANT)

We have learned there are essential attributes of a servant PD caregiver that we all should consider. I have given the name "PLS," which can be said as the "Please" method for ease of remembering. You are finding a way to please your loved one as you put your needs second.

"P" IS FOR PATIENCE

There are very few conditions more demanding of a caregiver than battling a slow degenerative disease process. Patients are living nearly an average life expectancy with PD; thus, for many caregivers, you are investing caregiving role for more than twenty years and sometimes even more than thirty years.

Also, the progressive slowness of individuals with PD is a real test on one's patience. It is much easier to push a more advanced patient in a wheelchair quickly down the walkway than to have to walk incredibly slow while your loved one attempts to shuffle along behind a walker. Some patients experience freezing of gait, which causes long pauses in which the patient is unable to initiate a gait or gets stuck in the most precarious places. A caregiver is tempted to just grab the patient and pull them along to speed up the process. Unfortunately, as we know, this doesn't work.

There is not just physical slowness but also mental slowness. A more advanced patient may take many long minutes to gather their thoughts and then articulate the response they wish to communicate. You might ask them a question and have to wait a long time for their response. If you are in a social setting, you might lose your patience and just speak for the patient or cut them off to hurry up the conversation for the sake of the other listeners.

A servant caregiver does everything in their power to be patient and let their loved one take their time getting dressed, walking down the aisle, out to the car, and finish the statement they were asked to provide. A servant caregiver knows that this is difficult to carry out in a real world setting, but they also know how important it is to maintain the dignity of the patient and to allow their loved one the chance to accomplish tasks without always having someone do it for them. If the person with PD requests assistance, then yes, the caregiver free to intervene on their behalf.

"L" IS FOR LEADERSHIP

As a servant caregiver for a PD patient, if you are not already the leader of the family, then you will undoubtedly take on the role of the leader. As the disease advances the patient will now defer to you as the decision-maker for everything. You will take over and manage the family finances. You will make the decisions for your household. You will organize the caregiving providers helping your loved one. You will oversee the records and keep the information organized.

This new role may be daunting to many caregivers who may have been in the reverse role most of their adult life. For instance, if a spouse was used to her husband managing the bills, taking care of the family taxes, making the decisions on investments and retirement funds, and organizing the health information for the family, these responsibilities may reverse after PD affects the family. Now the wife as a caregiver for her husband with PD may be faced with all of these tasks since her husband is no longer able to manage these jobs and make wise decisions. Now the wife either has to learn how to manage these areas or find trusted help from someone else to advise her.

In some cases, a family business may need to be managed, or new managers may need to be found since the patient is no longer able to participate in these business dealings. A family member who is now the caregiver may not have any knowledge or skills in understanding the business, let alone make wise decisions in the loved one's place.

The role of a family leader may be a difficult transition for some caregivers. However, the servant caregiver finds the resources and help needed to carry out this process to relieve the burden from the loved one with PD. In many cases, this is the safest move to make even before it may be absolutely time to transition leadership responsibilities. In particular, if medications and PD are causing an individual to make risky financial decisions or obsessed with spending money that may not be in the budget, then the caregiver needs to put safeguards in place to protect the family finances.

"S" IS FOR SERVANT

As a servant caregiver, we are putting our loved one's needs ahead of ourselves. This is quite difficult to do in reality for many individuals. Perhaps if the patient is a loved one or spouse, then this task is a more practical goal. But nevertheless, whether more or less practical, a caregiver for a loved one with PD should have as a goal to be a servant caregiver. If you are an adult child caring for your parent with PD, then your immediate priority may be the needs of your spouse and/or children. You will know best how to balance what is needed to serve the needs of the entire family.

If we keep the needs of our loved one as the top priority before our own needs, then we can achieve the full self-giving servant caregiving that helps the patient the most. I know what many are thinking about this. "What about my own needs? What about keeping myself healthy and attending to my needs?" These questions emerge from most books (including this one) and organizations telling caregivers that they must take time for themselves. Some resources advocate doing what is best for themselves over the needs of others. This book offers a way to balance caring for your loved one with PD *and* taking care of yourself.

Servant caregiving does not require the caregiver to abandon all care for themselves. The caregiver needs to have adequate sleep, nutrition, exercise, emotional support, cognitive stimulation, and spiritual time. The art of caregiving requires the caregiver to find ways to achieve a balance that is centered on others before self but not to the neglect of their self. This is a delicate balance and one that I myself struggle with every day in caring for my own mother.

I have seen the best caregivers in my practice leverage the "PLS" method over and over again, without knowing they were following a particular process. As I spoke to some of the most experienced caregivers who had been with their loved one through the entire battle with PD until, eventually, their loved one passed. The former caregiver would tell me how happy they were that they followed this type of caregiving method. They felt no guilt or shame afterwards. Although they thought they could have done a better job, we recognized that it could not have been humanly possible to be better caregivers than they were for their loved one with PD. These former caregivers were grateful to have had the opportunity to serve their family member all those years. Even in the difficult times and even in times when they did not get a thank you or any positive recognition, these former caregivers still found it was worth everything to be at the service of their family member who needed them during those desperate times. They would not have changed anything and now live in peace about their experience.

Now it is your turn to realize that you are doing a better job than you think! You may be doing all of these things discussed and not realize how important your steps have been in caring for your loved one. We all have the potential room for improvement. I pray that something in this book will help you along your journey caring for your loved one. "PLS" your loved one by adopting this method.

MORE CAREGIVER TO CAREGIVER RECOMMENDATIONS

Be THE expert in caring for the patient. You will get lots of advice, criticism, and thoughts about how to care for your loved one with PD. There are lots of resources available. However, YOU have to make the final decision. Trust your judgment. No one is living in your situation. No one knows your relationship like you do. No one knows the best ways to help your loved one. Be confident in what you are doing. This gives the patient comfort by feeling your confidence in what is going on.

The PD caregiver needs to come to terms with this new life assignment. This situation was not planned, was not asked for, but here it is. We need to accept the new role, achieve peace with it and decide to take it on the best we can. Any other approach will lead to more frustration, guilt, and poor quality of life for you and your family.

A loving caregiver is always a better caregiver. It is easy to get frustrated and easy to lash out at your loved one. If you remember each day that your job is to serve and to love, then you cannot go wrong. God commands us to love our neighbors as ourselves. Provide what is vital to the patient, not to yourself first. As a servant caregiver, if we do everything with a giving, loving heart, then this service will repay you in exponential ways. Holding resentment and anger at your situation and directing the emotion at the patient only leads to more frustration, guilt, and anger. Ultimately this negative cycle is bad for both of you.

Calmness is better for the PD patient because it will reduce symptoms and thus suffering. You will be more effective. You will enjoy life more, if you are not frustrated and second- guessing what you are doing or if doing it right. Look at your decisions and approaches as "Is it working?" Not is the decision or approach right or wrong. Use common sense. You can make sound judgments. You will make mistakes but that is ok if you learn from the mistakes. No one expects you to be perfect. There is no grade. Patients with PD are tough. The patients are dealing with a lot and have to learn how to handle difficult times. They can also manage your occasional mistakes. PD is unpredictable so just go with it and don't worry if you don't understand everything.

Don't blame yourself for the decisions you have to make. Don't feel guilty if you have to move your loved one into a facility or get outside help. It is ok. You are not a failure. You know when it is time to get help and don't second-guess your decision. Even if your children disagree on your approach or decisions, you are in charge, you are the expert, and you make the decisions as the primary caregiver. Don't be afraid to ask the patient, "How am I doing as a caregiver?

What am I doing that you don't like? Getting involved in local support groups and organizations can be very fulfilling. These new friends can be an excellent resource for both the caregiver and the patient. Education from the medical field is often a significant part of the support group meetings.

If you do not fit into one group, don't give up. Try some other groups, and you will likely find a good fit. If your loved one with PD doesn't want to go at this stage, consider going yourself to learn more and stay updated for both of you. Additionally, there are support groups online through several organizations and educational seminars that can also be helpful. These are usually free events. There may even be pharmaceutical company and device company representatives at the meeting to provide information about new therapies for PD or other therapy services such as Speech and Swallow Therapy or Physical Therapy or Occupational Therapy service available. Information about exercise groups and classes may also interest you.

The PD organization, both nationally and locally, provides many excellent services for patients from support groups to exercise classes. As a non-profit, the organization uses fundraisers to enable these programs and services. I always encourage patients and caregivers, along with other family members, to consider participating in the events that the organization hosts for fundraising. This is usually a walk/run event or another fundraising event that is an excellent opportunity to show support for your loved one while contributing to a great cause.

Patients love to see their family members all wearing the same t-shirt with their family team showing their love and support for them at the event. Many patients look forward to these events each year because the patient always feels better when they are helping other people and participating in an event larger than themselves. If they can set out, walk and run during the event, or play golf at the golf tournament fundraiser, it is a way to show that the disease is not getting the best of them, and they are actively fighting back!

PATIENTS ASSESS THEIR CAREGIVER

When we reviewed our research of caregivers and patients in the clinic, we asked all of the patients with PD to evaluate how they thought their caregiver was doing in caring for their needs. 100 percent of the patients filled out their responses independently, anonymously without the caregiver knowing the patient's response. The patients also knew that their response would not be shared with their loved ones.

In all cases where the caregiver did not feel like they were doing a good job taking care of their loved one with PD, the patient had the exact opposite evaluation. All of the patients felt that the caregiver was doing an excellent job. So if caregivers are concerned about anyone evaluating their caregiving ability, it should be the person with PD because this is ultimately the only person's opinion that matters. All caregivers are better caregivers than they themselves thought they were because the person with PD thought they were excellent caregivers despite the self-doubt and self-criticism that the caregiver expressed about themselves.

You know these things but it's helpful to hear it. We hope it helps you continue your caregiving journey with more peace and with the knowledge that your reward will ultimately await you, even if your days are thankless. Ultimately, you will be happier in serving others – your loved one – than in serving yourself.

CHAPTER 13

CONCLUSION

What legacy do you wish to leave for your family regarding how you performed as the Parkinson caregiver?

I am not referring to whether your loved one was pleased with your efforts, or that you did the best job of all the caregivers in your support group. I am curious about how the future generations of your family will look back with pride and loving thoughts about the example that you established in how to care for another loved one.

I believe that family members already recognize the great effort you are putting into caregiving. They appreciate the love that you show your loved one with PD and the absolute dedication that you give your loved one. They see the sacrifices you make daily.

When you envision the type of caregiving you provided your loved one, what do you see? What were your strengths as a caregiver? How about your weaknesses? Are there any aspects of your caregiving that you would like to change? How satisfied are you with the job you are doing? Does guilt factor into any negative feelings or thoughts that you have about your performance thus far?

I encourage you to take a few minutes right now to pause and consider the following question: "What does a successful caregiver for a PD patient look like to me?" As you think about this question, are you drawing a blank? As you think more about this question, what measurements are you using to evaluate the performance of a caregiver?

Some of our caregivers would answer this question in comparison to the other caregivers that they know around them. One might say, "Well, compared to the other men in the caregiving group, I certainly sacrifice more than they do."

Some caregivers may evaluate their performance based upon the fact that they have kept their loved one at home and not in a nursing care facility. A caregiver may say, "I only need help from the outside once a week while everyone else I know seems to need help every day."

The majority of the caregivers, however, report a negative evaluation of their performance of a caregiver. They are often overly hard on themselves and do not feel confident in the type of care they provided. They worry that they are not caregiving the "right way," and they worry that their caregiving may have caused more problems for the patient than help them.

There is no doubt that a caregiver has the most critical impact on the patient with PD. What impact do you want to have on your loved one's journey? You are most likely already making an impact by your love and empathy for your loved one. You might have realized through reading this book that there are some changes you would like to make to improve the impact of your caregiving. Your caregiving relationship can grow stronger, and your connection can provide even more relief from the suffering. You have the power to impact the course of the disease and to leave a legacy for your family for future generations to observe what actual caregiving means.

ENVISION A FUTURE

As a caregiver, imagine how you want to feel about your caregiving efforts someday in the future. It doesn't matter that you did everything exactly right along the way in taking care of your loved one's needs. Sure, there may have been better ways to handle certain situations. Will you be able to say to someone, "I know my loved one felt the love and compassionate care that I provided throughout the illness?" What would your loved one say about the kind of caregiving you offered over the years? Approach each day of caregiving with the end in mind. What is the legacy you want to leave on how you cared for your loved one?

Caregivers take on an enormous responsibility. They are now typically handling the home, possibly the family business, finances, bills. They become the sole decision maker for most items. They manage the health records for the patient as well as prescriptions. They also have to continue to monitor and maintain their own needs.

Caregivers find that they must be flexible. Parkinson's Disease is unpredictable, with many twists and turns. The symptoms are ever-changing. New problems present themselves at unpredictable times. There are constant changes and for many caregivers, they feel as if they are riding a rollercoaster. The patient may fluctuate in how they treat the caregiver, and how they act toward the caregiver. You might find that plans will change, often right before the event, and many trips may be canceled or rescheduled due to the disease.

You must have a servant heart. Patience is so important and it is easy to get irritated. You will likely not feel as appreciated as you would like. Patients are slow and take more time to perform tasks. Love the patient always. Enjoy giving more than receiving. Always think about what is important to the patient, respect their needs and wishes. Care with confidence and always remember that you are a better caregiver than you think!

John's Story

John has been a caregiver for his wife's twenty-six-year battle with PD. After her death, he shared with me many of his thoughts about the experience. John told me that he never imagined how stressful the caregiving would be due to PD. He said, "I was able to adjust to the physical demands of caring for her. However, I had the most difficulty dealing with the mental changes. I didn't realize how much her personality had changed over the years due to the illness. The effects the disease had on her memory, thinking skills, and judgment were devastating to me. She was slipping away from me every day and there was nothing I could do to fix the problem. The only thing I could do every day was to love her! Everything I did for her each and every day was an expression of love. No matter how many times I had to feed her, help her in and out of the bathroom, repeat the same answer to her question for the thirtieth time, all of my giving to her was an expression of my love for her. I vowed to her when we got married that I would take care of her, 'In sickness and in health.' And that is what I did."

John told me that there is not a day that goes by that he doesn't thank God for the time they had together and the love that they shared. He knows that he made plenty of mistakes along the way and could have done certain tasks better but he also knows that he could not have loved her any more than he did. He will be able to rest well each night knowing that he did his best in caring for her. Even during the times that she was unable to communicate to him her appreciation for the love and care that John provided, he knew that she could feel his love every day. And in the end that is all that matters. That is what caregivers are called to do. That is what you and I are called to do.

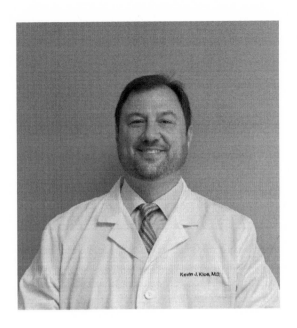

Kevin Klos, MD, is a board-certified Movement Disorder Specialist Neurologist and founder of the Movement Disorder Clinic of Oklahoma. He is a full time Parkinson's disease clinician as well as clinical trial researcher. He is a nationally recognized Parkinson's disease caregiver mentor and offers a weekly podcast for PD caregivers and families. Kevin and his wife Shannon make their home in Tulsa, Oklahoma along with their seven children, Gavin, Rosie, AJ, Felicity, Leo, Titus, and Callista.

Visit www.pdcaring.com for more information.